THE PRESIDENT IS
A SICK MAN

THE PRESIDENT IS
A SICK MAN

WHEREIN THE SUPPOSEDLY VIRTUOUS
GROVER CLEVELAND SURVIVES
A SECRET SURGERY AT SEA
AND VILIFIES
THE COURAGEOUS NEWSPAPERMAN
WHO DARED
EXPOSE THE TRUTH

MATTHEW ALGEO

CHICAGO
REVIEW
PRESS

Library of Congress Cataloging-in-Publication Data

Algeo, Matthew.

The president is a sick man : wherein the supposedly virtuous Grover Cleveland survives a secret surgery at sea and vilifies the courageous newspaperman who dared expose the truth / Matthew Algeo. — 1st ed.

p. cm.

Includes bibliographical references and index.

ISBN 978-1-56976-350-6 (hardcover)

1. Cleveland, Grover, 1837-1908—Health. 2. Cleveland, Grover, 1837-1908—Relations with journalists. 3. Depressions—1893—United States. 4. Bimetalism—United States—History—19th century. 5. United States—Politics and government—1893-1897. 6. Press and politics—United States—History—19th century. 7. Edwards, E. Jay (Elisha Jay), 1847-1924. I. Title.

E706.A54 2011

973.8'7092—dc22

2010044639

Interior design: Jonathan Hahn

Published by Chicago Review Press, Incorporated

814 North Franklin Street

Chicago, Illinois 60610

ISBN 978-1-56976-350-6

Printed in the United States of America

5 4 3 2

To Ann and Joan,
my sisters

Tell the truth.
— GROVER CLEVELAND

CONTENTS

PREFACE

O N JULY 1, 1893, Grover Cleveland, the president of the United States, vanished. He boarded a friend's yacht, sailed into the calm, blue waters of Long Island Sound, and—poof—he disappeared. Independence Day passed with the president's whereabouts unknown.

Grover Cleveland would not be heard from again for five days. What happened during those five days—and in the days, weeks, and months that followed—was so incredible that, even when the truth was finally revealed, many Americans simply could not believe it.

The President Is a Sick Man is about an extraordinary but almost unknown chapter in American history, about a brazen political cover-up that was as diabolical as—and infinitely more successful than—Watergate. It's about the lone reporter who uncovered the scandal, only to be branded a liar and "a disgrace to journalism." And it's about that reporter's belated vindication.

This book is also about life in the 1890s, and the echoes of the past that inform us today. The era's most controversial political issue was the money question: Should our currency be based on gold or silver? It may seem arcane to us today when our currency is based on, well, nothing more than the good faith of the federal government, but the gold-versus-silver debate grew so rancorous that it threatened to explode into a second Civil War. It also may have inspired a down-on-his-luck news-paper reporter named L. Frank Baum to write a children's book called *The Wonderful Wizard of Oz*, which many believe is an allegory for the money question.

In the following pages you will be introduced to the youngest First Lady in American history, a Rockefeller who sold patent medicines of questionable value, the doctor who performed one of the first success-ful brain surgeries in the United States, newspaper publishers uncon-strained by integrity, a cigarette-smoking tightrope walker, and a hand-ful of unfortunate suicides.

You will also meet Stephen Grover Cleveland, twice elected presi-dent of the United States, and a man so famously honest that perhaps his most memorable quotation is: "Tell the truth." But Grover Cleve-land was not as honest as he (or history) would have you believe. In fact, he was no less deceitful than any successful politician, and, in the sum-mer of 1893, he deceived the entire nation.

The facts concerning the disappearance of Grover Cleveland that summer were so well concealed that even today, more than a century later, a full and fair account has never been published. Until now.

What follows is a true story.

THE PRESIDENT IS
A SICK MAN

PART I

THE OPERATION

1

A ROUGH SPOT

MARCH 4, 1893, should have been a triumphant day for Grover Cleveland. After all, it was the day he was sworn in for an unprecedented second, nonconsecutive term as president. But when he awoke that morning, his emotions must have been mixed. Snow had fallen overnight, covering Washington in a frozen blanket. Gray skies threatened more. A cold wind rattled the windows of his suite at the Arlington Hotel on Vermont Avenue.

And the lousy weather was the least of his worries.

It was not an auspicious moment to assume the presidency, and Grover Cleveland knew it. "I hope the skies will lighten up by and by," he'd written a friend a few weeks earlier, "but I have never seen a day since I consented to drift with events that I have not cursed myself for yielding." He was about to take the reins of a nation teetering on the brink of chaos. The economy was in ruins. Unemployment was rampant. Stock prices were plummeting. Banks and factories were closing by the score. Just nine days earlier, the once mighty Reading Railroad had gone bankrupt. More and bigger businesses were sure to follow the Reading into insolvency. Foreign investors who had flooded the country with capital after the Civil War were retreating like Lee from Gettysburg.

The Panic of 1893 was underway. It would spawn the worst economic catastrophe in American history, unsurpassed until the Great Depression.

Cleveland, who was just two weeks shy of his fifty-sixth birthday, emerged from the hotel at eleven o'clock that morning and climbed into a gleaming black carriage for the short ride to the Executive Mansion.* Though he weighed nearly three hundred pounds, Cleveland moved with an easy grace that belied his massive girth. Just under six feet tall, nearly rectangular in shape, with thinning brown hair combed straight back and a big walrus moustache, Grover Cleveland was, figuratively and literally, the biggest political figure of his generation.

Wrapped in a long, black overcoat with a velvet collar, Cleveland rode the open carriage to 1600 Pennsylvania Avenue. There he called on President Benjamin Harrison. Four years earlier, their roles had been reversed: Cleveland was the outgoing president, Harrison the incoming. The two men spent a few minutes in the Blue Room discussing the transition and then climbed into another open carriage for the mile-long ride down Pennsylvania Avenue to the inauguration ceremony at the Capitol. On the way they chatted amiably about the weather. Eight years earlier, in 1885, the sun had shone so brightly on Cleveland's first inauguration that "Cleveland weather" became a national catchphrase for a sunny day. But there would be no Cleveland weather on this day, for, as one congressman recalled, the conditions were "as bad as mortal man ever endured, windy, stormy, sleety, icy."

When they reached the Capitol, Cleveland and Harrison went inside the Senate chamber for the swearing in of Vice President Adlai Stevenson. (Stevenson was the grandfather of the 1952 and 1956 Democratic presidential nominee of the same name.) Many dignitaries were delayed by the weather, and it was nearly one thirty—ninety minutes

---

* The president's residence would not come to be commonly known as the White House until Theodore Roosevelt's presidency (1901–1909).

late—before the festivities moved outside for Cleveland to take his own oath. A wooden platform draped with bunting had been erected at the bottom of the steps on the east side of the Capitol. About ten thousand people stood shivering on the frozen ground to watch the ceremony. Frances Cleveland, Grover's wildly popular wife, was one of the first to emerge from the Capitol. As soon as she appeared, a huge cheer went up—the loudest of the day, according to some observers. Frances took special care walking down the slippery marble steps to her seat on the platform, for, unbeknownst to anyone outside her family, the once and soon-to-be First Lady was two months pregnant.

Then came members of the outgoing and incoming cabinets, the nine Supreme Court justices, and assorted foreign diplomats in plumed hats. Finally, Harrison and Cleveland emerged, walking down the steps side by side. Harrison took his seat in a plush leather chair in the front row, while Cleveland removed his top hat and, without introduction or fanfare, walked up to the front of the platform. Snow had started fall-

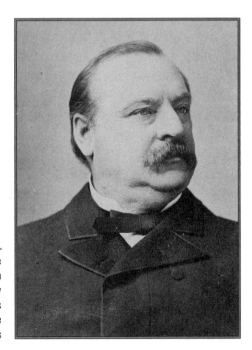

Grover Cleveland, photographed in 1888. Cleveland is the only president to have served two nonconsecutive terms. When he began his second term, the country was in the throes of an economic crisis that would come to be known as the Panic of 1893. LIBRARY OF CONGRESS

ing again. Cleveland held his hat in his left hand. Facing a sea of black umbrellas, he launched into his second inaugural address.

Cleveland was one of the most famous public speakers of his time. Befitting a man of his size, he had a booming voice—stentorian, as the papers liked to say. He once gave a speech to twenty thousand people at the old Madison Square Garden, and, it was reported, every single one of them could hear every single word. And he always delivered his speeches from memory, without so much as notes. His memory was said to be photographic. One newspaper reported that he could "repeat pages of poetry or of prose, after a single reading."

But even a bellowing Grover Cleveland could not overcome Mother Nature. Without the benefit of artificial amplification, his words were scattered by the howling wind. The speech lasted about twenty minutes. The frigid crowd barely heard a word of it.

Which is too bad, because, as inaugural speeches go, it wasn't half bad. He railed against "the waste of public money," and he gave one of the most unequivocal calls for civil rights that had ever been expressed in an inaugural, though it was expressed in his typically cumbersome way: "Loyalty to the principles upon which our government rests positively demands that the equality before the law which it guarantees to every citizen should be justly and in good faith conceded in all parts of the land. The enjoyment of this right follows the badge of citizenship wherever found, and, unimpaired by race or color, it appeals for recognition to American manliness and fairness."

Regarding the ruinous economy, which he delicately referred to as "our present embarrassing situation," he promised to do everything in his power to "avert financial disaster," but he also warned Americans not to expect a handout: "The lessons of paternalism ought to be unlearned and the better lesson taught that, while the people should patriotically and cheerfully support their Government, its functions do not include the support of the people."

Cleveland also made an interesting analogy, saying "it behooves us to constantly watch for every symptom of insidious infirmity that threatens our national vigor."

"The strong man who in the confidence of sturdy health courts the sternest activities of life and rejoices in the hardihood of constant labor may still have lurking near his vitals the unheeded disease that dooms him to sudden collapse."

After the speech, Chief Justice Melville Fuller rose and administered the oath of office, his black robe whipping in the wind. Cleveland put his hand on the same family Bible he'd been sworn in on eight years earlier, listened as Fuller read the oath, and then "assented" to it with a bow of his head. Cleveland bent down to kiss the Bible, which was opened to the ninety-first psalm: "With long life will I satisfy him, and shew him my salvation." As the newly inaugurated president turned to walk back into the Capitol, Frances suddenly stepped forward and kissed him tenderly on the cheek. It was a shocking display of public affection for the time, and the audience roared in surprise and delight. Amid great

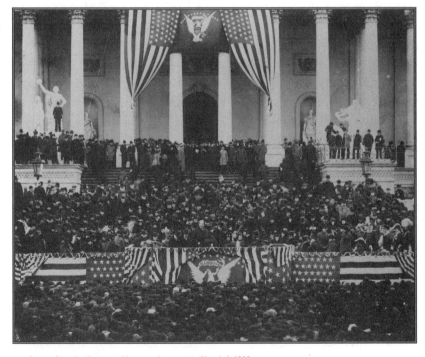

Grover Cleveland's second inaugural ceremony, March 4, 1893. LIBRARY OF CONGRESS

cheering, Cleveland, a tad embarrassed, walked up the steps of the east portico and into the Capitol.

That afternoon, Grover watched the inaugural parade from a reviewing stand in front of the White House, while Frances watched from inside a friend's apartment. More than twenty-five thousand people marched in the wind and snow, including thousands of Civil War veterans. The parade featured Buffalo Bill Cody and his Wild West show, as well as trained seals, acrobats, dancing horses, and dog acts. One marcher released a brown rooster in front of the reviewing stand as a gift for the Clevelands' seventeen-month-old daughter, Ruth. A contingent from the Army Corps of Engineers stopped in front of the president and released a dozen carrier pigeons bearing messages to be delivered to the Naval Academy in Annapolis ("Beat Navy," perhaps?).

The inaugural parade also included, for the first time, women.

It lasted more than four hours. By the time it was finally over, Grover's moustache was covered with frost, and the reviewing stand was dripping with icicles.

Yet for all the ceremony and spectacle, the mood in the capital that Inauguration Day was subdued, even somber. The bleachers that lined the parade route along Pennsylvania Avenue were half empty. The railroads estimated it was the lowest attended inaugural in memory. Disappointed vendors, laden with a dizzying array of Cleveland trinkets—badges, medallions, canes, handkerchiefs, balloons—couldn't give them away. The inaugural ball held that night at the Pension Office—now the National Building Museum—was so poorly attended that one newspaper declared it a "failure." The weather was partly to blame, of course, but so was the economy. Americans were in no mood to celebrate.

Underlying the financial crisis in 1893 was what was known, in the rather oblique vernacular of the day, as the money question. It was a question as old as mankind: What should represent value? In 1792 the United States Congress passed the Coinage Act, which defined one dollar as a coin containing 371.25 grains of pure silver. This put the fledgling nation on the silver standard, though the act also permitted the minting of gold coins and set the value of gold at fifteen times the value of silver. In 1834 the ratio was raised to sixteen to one. In other words, by law, sixteen ounces—one pound—of silver was worth the same as an ounce of gold.

During the Civil War, the U.S. Treasury began issuing paper banknotes in place of gold coins. These "gold certificates" were much cheaper to produce than coins, not to mention much easier to carry, and they could be redeemed for gold at the Treasury or one of its many branches, known as subtreasuries. This effectively put the country on the gold standard, and in 1873 Congress made it official by passing another Coinage Act, which "demonetized" silver. (The Treasury also experimented with fiat currency during the war. Those banknotes could not be redeemed for a metal but were still considered legal tender. It was an idea that took a while to catch on. But it did.)

Just in case anybody wanted to redeem their gold certificates, the Treasury kept an ample supply of gold on hand—at least $100 million. But as long as people had faith in the economy—and knew their gold was safe in a government vault and could, theoretically, be claimed at any time—everything was copasetic.

In 1877, U.S. gold production peaked at $46 million and then began a steady decline. The population, however, continued to grow, resulting in a "money famine": there wasn't enough cash to go around. Economists refer to this period in American history as the Great Deflation.

With gold production declining, mine operators turned to silver, and by 1890 silver production reached $57 million annually, far exceeding gold production. The most productive silver mines were in the Western states, and as those states began to enter the union (Nevada in 1864, Colorado in 1876, Montana in 1889) their representatives in Congress began to clamor for "bimetallism"—they wanted banknotes to be backed by silver as well as gold. In 1878 Congress passed the Bland-Allison Act, which required the Treasury to issue silver certificates for the first time. Twelve years later, in 1890, Congress passed the Sherman Silver Purchase Act, which required the federal government to buy a staggering 4.5 million ounces of silver every month and issue a commensurate amount of banknotes—notes that could be redeemed for either silver or gold. This dramatically increased the amount of money in circulation, resulting in rampant inflation.

Of course, Western silver mining interests didn't mind a little inflation. Nor did Southern and Midwestern farmers, who, after a string of poor crops, were heavily in debt. Now the money they paid their bills with was worth less than the money they'd borrowed. The "cheaper" money made it easier for them to pay their creditors. If you're in debt, inflation is good. If you're a lender, not so much.

And the lenders, by and large, were Eastern bankers and businessmen, who liked to call themselves "sound money men." They blamed silver—and the inflation it caused—for the nation's economic woes and their own diminishing fortunes. They wanted silver demonetized again and the nation categorically returned to the gold standard.

As new and larger silver veins were discovered, the financial situation deteriorated precipitously. While the value of silver to gold was set by law at sixteen to one, by the early 1890s the real value of silver to gold had plummeted to something closer to thirty-two to one. And, since silver certificates could be redeemed for either metal . . . well, you didn't have to be J. P. Morgan to figure out that you could double your money by exchanging fifty cents' worth of silver for a dollar in gold. It was legislated alchemy. Inevitably, the Treasury's gold supply began to dwindle, and, in April 1893, just a month after Cleveland began his second term, it dipped below the hugely symbolic $100 million mark for the first time; the panic that was gripping the nation only heightened.

The money question divided the nation more bitterly than any issue since slavery. It pitted Eastern "goldbugs" against Southern and Western "silverites." In pro-silver Kansas there was even talk of secession.

Compounding the financial crisis was a speculative bubble: railroads. Between 1870 and 1890, the number of miles of rail lines in the United States doubled to more than 120,000, while the population grew just 63 percent. The industry was hopelessly overbuilt. As a result, the railroads' freight charges plummeted—as did their profits. The Reading was only the first major railroad to go belly up in 1893. By the end of the year, the Erie, the Northern Pacific, the Union Pacific, and the Santa Fe would all collapse. In all, 119 railroads perished in 1893, and countless businesses that depended on those railroads simply vanished.

Grover Cleveland was a sound money man through and through, and he believed the only way to save the economy was to put the nation squarely back on the gold standard. "Manifestly nothing is more vital to our supremacy as a nation . . . than a sound and stable currency," he declared in his second inaugural—"a sound and stable currency" being code words for the gold standard.

Cleveland blamed the poor economy on the Silver Purchase Act, the law that required the government to purchase 4.5 million ounces of silver every month. He believed the act not only drained the government's gold reserves, it also undermined public confidence in the economy.

Cleveland had decided he would call a special session of Congress for the purpose of repealing the Silver Purchase Act. It only remained for him to decide when.

A political showdown was imminent.

———————⊸•••⊷———————

On the day after his inauguration, Grover Cleveland got down to business. His office was on the second floor of the White House, over the East Room. He sat behind a thirteen-hundred-pound oak desk made from the timbers of the British warship *Resolute*.* The working arrangements were, according to Cleveland's private secretary Robert Lincoln O'Brien, "of unbelievable simplicity." The president's entire staff comprised "seven white men, one white woman, and three colored messengers." The White House itself, O'Brien remembered, was "a Noah's Ark of every type of cockroach and water bug known to science."

But rather than tackling infinitely more momentous matters like the crumbling economy on his first full day back in office, Cleveland was

---

* The behemoth desk was a gift from Queen Victoria to President Hayes in 1880 and has been used by nearly every president since.

instead forced to deal with that scourge of nineteenth-century presidents: office seekers.

After President James Garfield was assassinated by a proverbial disappointed office seeker in 1881, Congress passed the Pendleton Act, which established the Civil Service Commission and began requiring some applicants for government jobs to pass written examinations demonstrating their abilities. But the law initially covered only a very small number of jobs. Even by the time Cleveland began his second term in 1893, civil servants filled just a quarter of the government's two hundred thousand jobs. The rest were still good-old-fashioned patronage jobs, to be filled as Cleveland chose. Cleveland supported civil service reform, but he was also a pragmatist. As the new party in power, Democrats were eager for their share of the spoils. Besides, patronage was a potent political weapon. Cleveland could grant or deny the power of patronage to members of Congress as he saw fit—and he would grant it only to those who promised to vote to repeal the Silver Purchase Act. About two weeks after taking office, Cleveland reached an agreement with Daniel Voorhees, a silver-leaning senator from Indiana and the chairman of the powerful Senate Finance Committee. The president gave Voorhees complete control of patronage in Indiana. In a letter to Cleveland dated March 20, Voorhees promised to return the favor. "You have indeed made me very deeply and permanently your debtor," Voorhees wrote, "and it will be one of the principal pleasures and purpose of my life, and at every opportunity, to recognize and justify, as far as may be in my power, the generous confidence and friendly regard you have extended to me."

Office seekers besieged President Cleveland, and rising unemployment only added to the crush. The boldest simply strolled through the front door of the White House, climbed a staircase covered with a threadbare carpet, and took a seat outside the president's office, in a crowded waiting room where the only diversion was a water cooler with an old jelly jar for a glass. Many applicants came armed with letters of recommendation from their congressmen. Each would be granted "an instant" to make his case, according to one observer. "Patiently listening to each request and making perfunctory response, the president then received the next and then the next, and no man of all that number who thus met him knew whether his plea had met with favor or refusal."

At times, the situation was farcical. Once, Vice President Stevenson called the Treasury to complain about an appointment, only to be told that he had written a letter of recommendation for the appointee. Unperturbed, the vice president admonished the department to ignore his written recommendations—only verbal recommendations were to be considered.

"The dreadful, frightful, damnable office seeking hangs over me, surrounds me," Cleveland lamented. It was, he said, a "nightmare." Yet, to some extent, he had only himself to blame. Other presidents routinely delegated the task of doling out jobs, especially the lesser posts, but Cleveland found it impossible to delegate authority. As his friend and erstwhile Democratic presidential candidate Samuel Tilden once noted, Cleveland was "the kind of man who would rather do something badly for himself than to have somebody else do it well." So Cleveland reviewed every application personally, even for the lowliest small town postmaster. More than a month after he started his second term, an acquaintance opined that the president had not been able "to give a moment's thought" to the money question because of the office seekers.

Meanwhile, the economy was only getting worse. On May 4, the National Cordage Company went bankrupt. The rope maker had once been a darling of investors. Just four months earlier it had paid a whopping 100 percent dividend. In reality, though, the company, like the railroads, was fatally overextended and deeply in debt. Its collapse sent Wall Street into another tailspin.

The next day, according to the *New York Times*, the floor of the stock exchange "might have passed for a morning in Bedlam."

That same day, May 5, Cleveland noticed for the first time a rough spot on the roof of his mouth. It was near his molars on the left side— his "cigar chewing side." He assumed it was nothing more serious than a minor dental problem, and given all he had on his plate at the time—the panic, the money question, the office seekers, Frances's pregnancy—it's

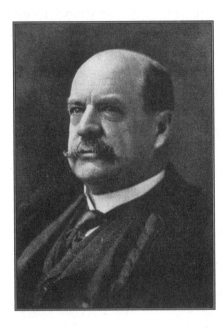

Joseph Decatur Bryant was a
prominent New York surgeon and
Grover Cleveland's close friend.
NATIONAL LIBRARY OF MEDICINE

hardly surprising he chose to ignore it. Accounts differ as to whether the
spot was painful, but by mid-June it had grown so large that it began
to worry the president deeply. As Frances recalled many years later, it
"often caused him to walk the floor at night." When Frances inspected
the spot, she saw what she described as a "peculiar lesion."

"I was alarmed when I saw it," Frances later wrote, "and felt that
Dr. Bryant who was our dear loyal friend and guide in all things medical should know it at once." Dr. Bryant was Joseph Decatur Bryant, a
prominent New York surgeon and the Cleveland family's physician.

"I wish very much to speak to you," Frances wrote Bryant in a letter
sent special delivery on Sunday, June 18, "especially about something
that the President has on the roof of his mouth." She requested that
they meet the next day at the railroad depot in Jersey City, New Jersey,
where Frances would be stopping on her way from Washington to Gray
Gables, the Clevelands' summer home on Cape Cod.

"Of course the request from Mrs. Cleveland was heeded," Bryant
later wrote, "and from her something of the physical characteristics of

the growth and her great anxiety regarding it were ascertained." Bryant agreed to go to Washington to examine the president.

Meanwhile, the White House physician, an army doctor named Robert M. O'Reilly, had already inspected the president's mouth. O'Reilly, who had been alerted to the lesion by the president's dentist, expressed "deep concern" over what he saw. He scraped a specimen and, without identifying the patient, sent it to the army laboratory for analysis. The pathologist there, Dr. William Welch, later remembered how he was told that "it was the most important specimen ever submitted for my examination and . . . to use the utmost diligence and skill." Welch, who suspected the specimen might have come from the president, determined that it was probably from a case of epithelioma, known today as squamous cell carcinoma.

In other words, a malignant tumor.

Dr. Bryant arrived in Washington on Thursday, June 22, and examined the president early the next morning. The physician saw "an ulcerated surface with an oval outline about the size of a quarter of a dollar extending from the inner surfaces of the molar teeth to within a quarter of an inch of the median line of the roof of the mouth and encroaching somewhat on the anterior part of the soft palate." One of Bryant's specialties happened to be oral tumors, and what he saw concerned him greatly. "To one familiar with the macroscopical appearances of epithelial growths," Bryant wrote, "no reasonable doubt could exist in his mind regarding the certainty of the malignant nature of this." (Epithelial cells are those that cover the surfaces and cavities of the body.)

"What do you think it is, Doctor?" Grover asked after the examination.

"It is a bad looking tenant," Bryant answered. "Were it in my mouth I would have it removed at once."

2

BIG STEVE

G ROVER CLEVELAND never gave much thought to his ancestry. He was, he once wrote, "very busy in an attempt to fulfill the duties of life without questioning how I got into the scrape." But his pedigree was more distinguished than he probably even knew. His great-great-grandfather and his great-grandfather, both named Aaron Cleveland, were famous Protestant ministers in colonial New England and New York. The younger Aaron's grandson, Richard Cleveland—Grover's father— was born in Norwich, Connecticut, in 1804. After graduating from Yale in 1824, Richard moved to Baltimore, where he studied theology. It was there that he met Ann Neal, the pretty daughter of a bookseller named Abner Neal. They were married in 1829.

Like his illustrious ancestors, Richard pursued a career in the pulpit. Unlike them, he found little success. He was never called to a prestigious church, and he never rose to a high position in his profession. Not a single word of any of his sermons was recorded for posterity. Some believed he was too humble for his own good. "He didn't have push enough," remembered one relative.

In November 1834, Richard Cleveland was called to serve as the minister at the Presbyterian church in Caldwell, New Jersey, about fifteen miles outside New York City. On March 18, 1837, Stephen Grover Cleveland was born in the Caldwell manse. Named for Stephen Grover, Richard's predecessor in the Caldwell pulpit, he was Richard and Ann's fifth child. Four more would follow. In 1841, Richard was called to Fayetteville, a small town near Syracuse in upstate New York.

Chubby, with bright blue eyes and light brown hair, Steve Cleveland was a friendly child who loved outdoor pursuits—swimming and fishing in the summer, hunting and sledding in the winter. According to neighbors he was "chuck full of fun," and not averse to occasional pranks, such as ringing the school bell in the middle of the night. In the classroom, he distinguished himself by hard work, not brilliance. "He considered well, and was resourceful," his sister Mary remembered, "but as a student Grover did not shine." In the words of his biographer Allan Nevins, young Steve was not—and never would be—a great intellectual force.

Money was tight in the Cleveland household, where there were eleven mouths to feed on a minister's salary. Young Steve did his part by working odd jobs. Fayetteville was near the Erie Canal, and when one of the village's lime quarries needed an empty barge, Steve would hail one and direct it to the quarry, a service for which he was reimbursed ten cents. To preempt competitors, Steve rose at four in the morning.

On October 1, 1853, when Steve was sixteen, his father died of peritonitis, an abdominal infection. Ann was left to care for the four youngest children. It was incumbent upon Steve to help support the family, and collecting dimes for hailing barges would not suffice. Later that fall, he abandoned his studies and moved to New York City, where he taught reading, writing, arithmetic, and geography at the New York Institute for the Blind. The institute was archetypically Dickensian, cold and dreary, with dreadful food and a loathsome headmaster named T. Colden Cooper. The 116 unfortunate inmates, ranging in age from eight to twenty-five, had been remanded there, often involuntarily, by county officials throughout the state.

In the fall of 1854, Cleveland quit his job at the institute, presumably without regrets. The following May, when he was eighteen, he went seeking fame and fortune in one of the boomtowns of the burgeoning Midwest: Cleveland, Ohio, a city that had been founded by a distant relative named Moses Cleaveland (supposedly, a mapmaker's error resulted in the spelling discrepancy). But he only made it as far as Buffalo, where he visited an uncle named Lewis Allen, who offered him room, board, and ten dollars a month to work on a Shorthorn cattle herd book that Allen was compiling. Steve accepted the offer.

Founded around 1800, Buffalo was a young city when Cleveland arrived. The children of its first white settlers still walked the streets, and they remembered well how the British had burned the city to the ground during the War of 1812. After the Erie Canal was completed in 1825, Buffalo became a boomtown, for it was where the canal joined the Great Lakes. From crops headed east to heavy equipment going the other way, everything passed through Buffalo. Between 1830 and 1860, the city's population grew tenfold, from eight thousand to eighty thousand.

And, like most boomtowns, it was a pretty wild place, teeming with brothels, saloons, and gambling halls. An old canalhand named E. E. Cronk later estimated that "sixty percent of the buildings on both sides of Canal Street from Erie Street to Commercial were houses of prostitution, thirty percent were saloons, and ten percent grocery stores, etc."

Not surprisingly, it was a dangerous place, too. Police patrolled Canal Street in threes: one in front, two in back. When the canal was dredged every spring, it wasn't unusual for eight or more human bodies to be discovered.

The canal itself was a frothing, stinking bouillabaisse of garbage, human and animal waste, agricultural and industrial runoff, and offal, not to mention the human corpses. The effluent occasionally produced giant methane bubbles that rose to the surface and exploded, unleashing a stench so foul it sickened some people for days. Disease was rampant. Periodic outbreaks of typhus, typhoid fever, and smallpox killed hundreds annually.

Yet, for all its faults—and there were many—Buffalo was also an exciting, vibrant, bustling place, filled with limitless opportunities for a young man with dreams and potential. There were fortunes to be made. You could have some fun there, too. One can imagine eighteen-year-old Stephen Grover Cleveland strolling down Canal Street's wooden sidewalks for the first time, smelling the fetid canal, hearing the beckoning calls of the ladies of the evening and the rollicking piano music emanating from the saloons. It must have enthralled the minister's son from Fayetteville. He resolved to stay in Buffalo.

Steve ended up living with his uncle and working on the herd book for a year. In his spare time he went fishing on the Niagara River, picked cherries in his uncle's orchard, and attended a fair in Utica. He also met some of his uncle's influential friends, including Henry W. Rogers, a principal in the prominent Buffalo law firm of Rogers, Bowen, and Rogers. Rogers was impressed by Steve and offered him a position at the firm as an office clerk. In his spare time, Steve would be allowed to study law in the firm's library; in essence, he would teach himself how to be a lawyer. This practice, called "reading law," was how lawyers often were trained until law schools became common in the 1890s. On Steve's first morning at the firm, Rogers tossed a copy of Blackstone's *Commentaries* on the young man's desk and told him dryly, "That's where they all begin." When the partners went out for lunch later that day, they forgot about Steve and locked him in the office. "Someday I will be better remembered," he promised himself.

Steve rented a cheap room in a boardinghouse near the firm and threw himself into his studies with a zeal that bordered on the obsessive, often reading until two or three in the morning.

It seems Steve had just two pastimes outside work. One was politics. In the fall of 1858, Cleveland, now twenty-one and old enough to vote, began volunteering for the local Democratic Party. Mostly he just helped get out the vote on Election Day. Why, precisely, he chose to become a Democrat is a bit of a mystery. As an old man he would say it was because the Democrats represented "greater solidity and conservatism" than the fledgling Republican Party. But it also might have had something to do with the fact that the three partners at Rogers, Bowen, and Rogers were all committed Democrats.

Steve's other pastime was partying. On those nights he wasn't staying up late reading law, he often patronized the saloons along Canal Street, where he could be found with a cigar in his mouth and a frothing mug of beer in his hand, leading his working-class German and Irish friends in bawdy songs. His favorite haunts were Diebold's, Schwabl's, Gillick's, and Louis Goetz's. On hot summer nights, he was likely to be spotted at Schenkelberger's or one of the city's other German beer gardens, where sawdust covered the floor and not much covered the pretty young fräuleins who kept his stein filled. Sometimes, he later admitted, his carousing would cause him to "lose a day." He was, generally speaking, a happy drunk, though he had a notoriously short temper that occasionally erupted. One night he was arguing politics with an acquaintance named Mike Falvey. The argument escalated into fisticuffs and ended when Cleveland "knocked Falvey into the gutter" on Seneca Street. Afterward the combatants patched things up over beers at Gillick's. In the opinion of his straitlaced uncle, Lewis Allen, Grover spent far too much time with "queer folk."

It was as if he had a split personality. There was the dour, disciplined law student and the fun-loving party animal. "There were always two Clevelands," writes Allan Nevins. "To the end of his life his intimates were struck by the gulf which separated the exuberant, jovial Cleveland of occasional hours of carefree banter, and the stern, unbending Cleveland of work and responsibility, whose life seemed hung round by a pall of duty."

In May 1859, after three and a half years of study, Stephen Grover Cleveland was admitted to the bar by the New York Supreme Court. He was twenty-two. Around this time, he decided to start going by Grover instead of Steve. As a law clerk he'd begun signing his name S. Grover Cleveland. Then he dropped the "S" altogether. Legend has it that he wanted his name to sound "more sonorous and distinctive." But to his family and to his friends in Buffalo, he would always remain Steve.

Grover stayed on at Rogers, Bowen, and Rogers, and was soon earning more than a $1,000 a year at a time when the average workingman was making only about $400.

In October 1862, an elderly Democrat named Cyrenius Torrance was elected Erie County district attorney. Cleveland was asked to be his assistant. It meant a big pay cut—the position paid just $500 a year—but Grover did not hesitate to accept the offer. He had decided to pursue a career in politics and regarded the position as a launching pad.

By now the Civil War was in its full fury, and in July 1863, Cleveland was drafted. That he was a loyal Unionist is indisputable; he was a "War Democrat" and may have even voted for Lincoln in 1864. But—occasional street fights notwithstanding—Cleveland had no stomach for battle, and the cause did not excite him. His position on slavery was ambiguous. Perhaps it was his Maryland-born mother's influence, but Grover was not known to be an ardent abolitionist.

Besides, he was still supporting his mother and two younger sisters, one of whom was now in college. Of his three brothers, one was already serving in the Union Army, and another had just been mustered out. Neither could afford to send money home. The third was a poorly paid Presbyterian minister. In Grover's opinion, military service was not an option. And there was a way out.

The Conscription Act of March 3, 1863, permitted draftees to avoid service by either furnishing a substitute or paying a "commutation fee" of $300. It was, inevitably, a controversial provision. Most workingmen could not afford to hire a substitute or pay the fee, which amounted to roughly 75 percent of their annual wages. German and Irish laborers were particularly aggrieved. They saw little to be gained by fighting for the freedom of the slaves, many of whom, they felt, would only come north and compete with them for jobs.

The Conscription Act stoked racial animosities that flared into violence in several Northern cities. In Buffalo, a white mob savagely beat and killed two African Americans in rioting on July 6, 1863. (Coincidentally, John Wilkes Booth was in town that week, performing at the Metropolitan Theatre.) In New York City a week later, a white mob burned a black orphanage to the ground. The orphans escaped with their lives, fortunately, but at least 120 other people in the city were killed over several days of rioting.

Instead of paying the $300 commutation fee to get out of the draft, Grover Cleveland found a substitute, a Great Lakes sailor named George Benninsky (or Brinske). Benninsky was an illiterate Polish immigrant who had come to the United States in 1851. Cleveland was acquainted with him through a friend named George Reinhart. Benninsky agreed to be Cleveland's substitute for $150, which was the going rate for substitutes in Buffalo at the time. It was a perfectly legal transaction. In fact, as Cleveland himself later pointed out, he could have paid much less. "Indeed," he wrote, "being then the assistant district attorney of Erie County, I had abundant opportunity to secure without expense a substitute from discharged convicts and from friendless persons accused of crime if I had wished to do so." On July 6, 1863—the day of the Buffalo draft riots—George Benninsky enlisted in the Seventy-Sixth New York. Years later, there would be rumors that Benninsky had suffered horrors in Cleveland's stead, but the truth is prosaic. After serving briefly and uneventfully at Rappahannock, Benninsky hurt his back. He spent the rest of the war as an orderly in Washington military hospitals.

Cleveland's elderly boss did not run for reelection in 1865, and Cleveland, as expected, won the Democratic nomination for district attorney. His Republican opponent was Lyman K. Bass, who happened to be one of Cleveland's drinking buddies—and his roommate. For the campaign they mutually pledged that each would imbibe no more than four glasses of lager daily. But one night they exceeded their allowance, and Bass proposed they "anticipate" their future allotment. "Grover," Bass said at the end of the night, "do you know we have anticipated the whole campaign?" The next night Grover produced two huge tankards to stand in for their glasses.

Democratic papers confidently predicted Cleveland's victory. "He is a young man, who, by his unaided exertions, has gained a high position at the bar, and whose character is above reproach," the *Buffalo*

Courier said. "He will be supported by hundreds of Republicans on these grounds."

But it was not to be. Cleveland carried the city's German and Irish wards, but Bass trounced him in the Yankee suburbs. Cleveland lost the election, though Bass probably picked up the tab for beers on election night.

Cleveland returned to private practice. Among his law partners at this time was Oscar Folsom, a former assistant U.S. attorney who was Cleveland's closest friend. The two men were nearly identical in age and temperament, hard workers who enjoyed a not infrequent tipple. When Folsom's daughter Frances was born in 1864, Cleveland had bought her a baby carriage and doted on her as if she were his own.

In 1870, Cleveland ran as the Democratic nominee for Erie County sheriff. It was a curious decision, for the position was not especially prestigious. But Grover was itching to get back into politics. He won the election by just 303 votes.

It was, in many ways, a thankless job. Buffalo was still a very rough place, and Grover was occasionally obliged to incarcerate acquaintances from the saloons he still frequented, albeit more discreetly. He was also obliged to carry out hangings, a task he found distasteful in the extreme. Though he did not oppose capital punishment, he was not by temperament vengeful or bloodthirsty. His mother urged him to assign a deputy to pull the lever that released the trapdoor underneath the condemned, as he easily could have done, but he said he could assign no man such a "hateful task." On the two occasions it was required, he pulled the lever himself.

As sheriff, Cleveland cracked down on graft. He personally measured the amount of firewood delivered to the jail, ensuring that it was the contracted quantity. He inspected the flour and oatmeal to ensure that it was of sufficient quality. He came to be known as incorruptible.

Cleveland won high praise for his performance as sheriff, but when his term ended in 1873, he did not run for reelection. Perhaps he found some of the obligations of the office too unseemly. In any event, he seems to have abandoned his dreams of a political career. Now thirty-six, he returned to the practice of law. His office was on the second floor of the Weed Block, an ugly building on the corner of Main and Swan Streets. Though he had amassed considerable savings by now and easily could have afforded a mansion in the suburbs, he still lived in a small apartment in the center of the city.

He specialized in civil litigation, and over the years his reputation grew. One of his clients was Standard Oil. In the courtroom he was methodical, never showy. His goal was not merely victory but a fair and just outcome for all parties. One colleague said he radiated a "quintessential integrity" and "everybody felt it." One judge before whom Cleveland argued many cases said he was "an exceedingly dangerous antagonist." It came to be widely assumed that Cleveland himself would someday ascend to the bench—perhaps even a seat on the state supreme court.

Grover continued to enjoy Buffalo's boisterous nightlife. Two or three nights a week he could still be found inside in a saloon. He never cooked for himself, instead taking all his meals in restaurants or rooming houses. German food was his favorite. Though he remained a Presbyterian, clearly he was not a rabid one. On a given Sunday he was more likely to be found in a pool hall than a pew. Years later he would cheerfully admit of his Buffalo years that he "had not been a saint." Still a bachelor, he was discreet about his romantic interests and kept his distance from the city's belles. He told his sisters he thought of getting married "a good many times." "And the more I think of it," he continued, "the more I think I'll not do it." Another time he told his sisters, rather cryptically, "I'm only waiting for my wife to grow up."

In all his years in Buffalo, Grover is known to have had just one serious relationship. It was with a vivacious and intelligent department store clerk named Maria Crofts Halpin. Maria was a thirty-three-year-old widow when she moved to Buffalo in 1871. She spoke French, attended one of the city's upper-class churches, and, as Allan Nevins delicately puts it, "she accepted the attentions of several men"—including Grover.

On September 14, 1874, Halpin gave birth to a son, whom she named Oscar Folsom Cleveland. Halpin identified Cleveland as the father. Cleveland, then thirty-seven, single, and well employed, did not admit paternity but did agree to provide for the child. The curious name that Halpin gave the baby—Oscar Folsom was Grover's law partner and best friend, after all—seems to suggest that she herself wasn't certain who the father was. One theory holds that Folsom was the father, but, since he was married, Halpin named Cleveland, hoping he would propose to her. And if Folsom was the father, the theory goes, Cleveland agreed to accept responsibility for the child to spare his friend the embarrassment and scandal of an unintended and illegitimate son. In any event, Cleveland did not propose marriage, and Halpin was left to raise the child alone. She began drinking heavily and was committed to an asylum for the "mentally deranged." The child was sent to an orphanage, and Cleveland, true to his word, paid the bill: five dollars a week.

After she was released from the asylum, Halpin unsuccessfully attempted to regain custody of the child. In desperation she kidnapped him from the orphanage. The child was soon recovered and eventually was adopted by a well-to-do family. Maria Halpin left Buffalo and remarried. (According to Nevins, the child grew up to become a "distinguished professional man," though other reports suggest he drank himself to death at an early age. His identity has never been publicly disclosed, but if he has any living descendents, DNA testing might clear up the lingering paternity question once and for all.)

Naturally, what Grover referred to as his "woman scrape" was the subject of much gossip in Buffalo, and once he became a national figure, it was inevitable that the story would surface in the papers.

Less than a year after the birth of the Halpin baby, Oscar Folsom was killed in a gruesome accident. He was returning home from a friend's house when his buggy collided with a wagon that was parked in front of a saloon on Niagara Street. Folsom was thrown to the ground and crushed under the wheels of his buggy. He suffered a fractured skull and massive internal injuries. Less than two hours later, he died. He was thirty-seven. Cleveland was working in his apartment when he heard the news that his best friend was dead. He could hardly believe it, and it would take him a long time to recover from the loss. Cleveland was named the executor of Folsom's estate, and he came to feel a special obligation to Folsom's widow and her eleven-year-old daughter Frances.

By the time he was forty, Grover's fondness for beer and bratwurst had begun to affect his physique. His weight approached 250 pounds, and his friends called him Big Steve. His nieces and nephews nicknamed him Uncle Jumbo. Self-assured as he was, neither moniker troubled him in the least. His only sources of exercise were hunting and fishing, pursuits he considered almost religious; true sportsmen, he believed, "appreciate the goodness of the Supreme Power who has made and beautified Nature's abiding-place." He didn't even like to walk, a task he considered "among the dreary and unsatisfying things in life." He joined the Beaver Island Club, an outdoor sports club on an island in the Niagara. On some outings he brought along chubby little "Frankie" Folsom, his late friend's daughter.

It was a comfortable life, and Cleveland seemed content.

———

At noon on March 4, 1881, James Garfield was sworn in as president, continuing a Republican stranglehold on the White House that stretched back to Lincoln's first inauguration twenty years earlier. It was a Thursday, so Grover Cleveland was undoubtedly hard at work. That night he might have read newspaper reports of the inauguration at one of his favorite watering holes. Still a loyal Democrat but disengaged from party politics, he fervently longed for the day that a Democrat would return to the White House. He could not have imagined—no one could have imagined—that, in exactly four years, a Democrat would return to the White House and that it would be Grover Cleveland himself.

In those four years Cleveland was swept up in a whirlwind that carried him, sometimes reluctantly, from the pleasant obscurity of his Buffalo law practice to the unimaginable pressures of the highest office in the land. His rise was more rapid and unlikely than that of any other chief executive. It was attributable, of course, to Cleveland's personal and political skills. But it was also attributable to the fact that, as Allan

Nevins puts it, "the stars were with him." Garfield was assassinated and died after just two hundred days in office, reconfiguring the political landscape in ways that would prove advantageous to Cleveland. And by the next presidential election, Cleveland himself would be a figure of national renown.

By 1881, Buffalo's municipal government had grown unconscionably corrupt. Aldermen openly accepted kickbacks for city contracts. A succession of mayors, both Republicans and Democrats, merely turned a blind eye. Voters were outraged. After the Republicans nominated a business-as-usual candidate for mayor, the Democrats began fishing around for an "aggressively honest" candidate. Many were considered before Cleveland, but none was willing to sacrifice his career for a position that paid just $2,500 annually (and in which he was not expected to profit from graft). Cleveland, who had amassed savings in excess of $70,000, could afford to run, and he had a reputation for unshakable honesty. He was arguing a case before Judge Albert Haight when a committee of Democratic officials interrupted the proceedings to formally offer Cleveland the nomination. Cleveland approached the bench.

"This is a committee from the Democratic city convention," he said to Haight, "and they want to nominate me for mayor. . . . What shall I do about it?"

"The mayoralty is an honorable position," answered the judge. "You're an old bachelor. You haven't any family to take care of. I'd advise you to accept."

Cleveland took the judge's advice. In his letter of acceptance he wrote, "Public officials are trustees of the people." A reporter later paraphrased Cleveland: "Public office is a public trust." It would become his mantra.

Cleveland won the election with 57 percent of the vote.

Once in office, Cleveland vetoed so many wasteful spending bills that he came to be known as the veto mayor. Most famously he vetoed a street-cleaning contract that would have gone to the highest bidder, a firm that bid $422,500—$109,000 more than the next highest bid. The difference, presumably, was to be divided among the aldermen. In his veto message, Cleveland called the contract "a most bare-faced, impudent, and shameless scheme to betray the interests of the people, and to worse than squander the public money." It was the kind of plain talk that would come to characterize Cleveland's political career. Indeed, as mayor, Cleveland's political persona burst into full flower. He was blunt, outspoken, honest. And he exuded a peculiar charisma. With his massive physique and booming voice, he seemed larger than life. Yet there was also something almost delicate about him. "In his movements Mr. Cleveland is deliberate, dignified, and graceful," the *New York Times* said of the mayor.

Cleveland was also instrumental in the construction of a new sewer system that diverted waste from the Erie Canal. This put an end to Buffalo's unappealing stench and dramatically improved public health.

The demands of his new office proved so unrelenting that Grover was finally forced to curb his partying. To the dismay of his friends on Canal Street, he was seen less and less.

In May 1882, Charles W. McCune, the editor of the *Buffalo Courier*, told a meeting of the Democratic State Committee that Grover Cleveland would make a fine candidate for governor. In an editorial the following month, the *Buffalo Sunday Times* said the same thing. By August, Cleveland had suddenly emerged as one of the leading contenders for the nomination.

Again, the stars were with him. At the nominating convention, two Democratic factions were deadlocked. Backed by a third, reformist wing of the party, Cleveland emerged as the compromise candidate and was nominated on the third ballot. The Republicans, meanwhile, nominated a typical machine politician. In frustration, Republicans who favored reform flocked to Cleveland.

On November 7, 1882, Cleveland was elected governor of New York with 58 percent of the vote. His star was rising so rapidly that even Cleveland himself could hardly believe it. In a letter written to his brother William on the night he was elected, Grover sounds as if he wondered what he'd gotten himself into: "The thought that has troubled me is, Can I perform my duties, and in such a manner as to do some good to the people of the state? I know there is room for it. . . . I know that I am honest and sincere in the desire to do well, but the question is whether I know enough to accomplish what I desire."

In the same letter, Grover also wrote, "I shall have no idea of reelection or any higher political preferment in my head, but be very thankful and happy if I can well serve one term as the people's governor."

In Albany, the veto mayor became the veto governor. He vetoed a bill that would have lowered fares on New York City's elevated railroad from ten cents to five cents. Understandably, the bill had broad popular support, but Cleveland believed it to be patently unconstitutional. The state and the railroad had entered into a contract that clearly permitted the railroad to set fares. The night he vetoed the bill, Cleveland went to bed believing that when he woke up the next morning he would be "the most unpopular man in the state of New York." Instead, the veto was hailed as an act of uncompromising political courage.

He was, fundamentally, a reformer. In challenging the spoils system, he took on Tammany Hall, the powerful New York City political machine. Pledging to "work for the interests of the people of the state, regardless of party or anything else," he insisted on hiring only the most qualified applicants for state government jobs. For superintendent of public works, he appointed a professional engineer, not a politician. For superintendent of insurance—a plum political position—Cleveland promoted the assistant superintendent instead of appointing a politician. After one round of appointments was announced, a Tammany official complained, "Out of all the three hundred places . . . Tammany was not guaranteed so much as a night watchman at Castle Garden." (Castle Garden was New York City's immigration center before Ellis Island.)

Governor Cleveland also forged an unlikely alliance with an up-and-coming Republican lawmaker named Theodore Roosevelt. At the time Roosevelt was twenty-three, his boyish face partly obscured by the massive sideburns that were then fashionable. When Roosevelt managed to push a civil service reform bill through the legislature, Cleveland was happy to sign it.

Grover was never afraid to confront the powerful, a quality that endeared him to voters. It was said he was loved for the enemies he made. When he refused to appoint to his staff a friend of Charles A. Dana, the influential publisher of the *New York Sun*, Dana was enraged. It was a slight that Dana would never forget, and it made him Cleveland's lifelong enemy.

Shortly after arriving in Albany, Cleveland hired Daniel S. Lamont as his private secretary. Lamont was a twenty-eight-year-old reporter for the *Albany Argus*. He'd met Cleveland during the gubernatorial campaign, and the two men hit it off immediately. "Lamont is a wonderful man," Cleveland once told a friend. "I never saw his like. He has no friends to gratify and no enemies to punish." Lamont, one reporter noted, was "discreet, industrious, and loyal . . . and capable of quite as hard work as Mr. Cleveland himself." Although Lamont was fourteen years younger than Cleveland, he would become one of his closest friends since Oscar Folsom. Lamont's vast knowledge of New York state politics was invaluable to the inexperienced governor, who had come to Albany a babe in the Empire State's political woods. In gratitude,

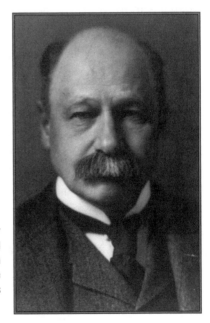

Dan Lamont was a twenty-eight-year-old reporter for an Albany newspaper when Grover Cleveland hired him to be his private secretary. The two men became close friends, and Lamont would become Cleveland's most trusted adviser. LIBRARY OF CONGRESS

Cleveland appointed Lamont an honorary colonel in the New York National Guard, and thereafter the former newspaperman would be known as Colonel Lamont—though Grover still called him Dan. For the rest of Cleveland's political career, Lamont would serve as his right-hand man, often acting as his press secretary and spokesman in the days before such positions were formalized.

The workload in Albany was crushing. On most nights, Cleveland and Lamont would work in the governor's office until midnight or later, when Cleveland would customarily announce, "Well, I guess we'll quit and call it half a day." The grueling schedule did not escape the notice of Albany residents, who were not accustomed to seeing governors burn the midnight oil. It worried them. "Plainly he is a man who is not tak-ing enough exercise," the *Albany Evening Journal* wrote three months into Cleveland's term. "There was not a night last week that he departed from the new Capitol before one a.m. Such work is killing work." Even Cleveland knew he was working too hard. "My head a good deal of the time doesn't feel right," he confessed to a friend in April.

There was, of course, even less time for carousing than when he was mayor of Buffalo. Besides, he was now in a strange town with few friends. His free time was spent mostly at the governor's mansion—the first house Cleveland lived in as an adult. He installed a pool table but otherwise made no major alterations. Still, it was impossible for him to curb his vices entirely. He continued to smoke cigars and enjoy occa-sional beers. And on Sunday afternoons he often played poker with a twenty-five-cent limit. "My father used to say that it was wicked to go fishing on Sunday," he would say, "but he never said anything about draw-poker."

Grover Cleveland's reputation began to extend beyond the borders of New York State, and in the spring of 1884, just over a year after becoming governor, his name was being mentioned as a possible Demo-cratic presidential candidate. Publicly, Cleveland professed no interest in the office. Privately, however, he began to marshal support for a bid. Clearly he had reconsidered the pledge he had made to his brother the night he was elected governor.

Yet again, the stars were with Grover Cleveland.

After James Garfield was assassinated, Chester Arthur became president. Arthur had been a notorious spoilsman, but as president he did a one-eighty and championed civil service reform. This infuriated Republican Party bosses, and instead of nominating Arthur for a full term in 1884, the Republicans chose James G. Blaine of Maine. It was a poor choice (though, had Arthur been nominated, he would not have survived another term anyway). Blaine, a former House speaker, senator, and secretary of state, was far from squeaky clean. Eight years earlier, he had been accused of accepting $100,000 from a railroad in exchange for favorable legislation.

When the Democrats convened a month after the Republicans, they were determined to nominate a reform-minded candidate to oppose Blaine. Cleveland, with his unimpeachable reputation and winning track record, was nominated overwhelmingly on just the second ballot.

Just ten days later, on July 21, 1884, the *Buffalo Telegraph* published an account of the Maria Halpin affair under the headline "A Terrible Tale; A Dark Chapter in a Public Man's History."

"A child was born out of wedlock," the story began. "Now ten years of age, this sturdy lad is named Oscar Folsom Cleveland. He and his mother have been supported in part by our ex-mayor, who now aspires to the White House. Astute readers may put the facts together and draw their own conclusions." The story was written not by a reporter but by George Ball, a Baptist minister in Buffalo and longtime thorn in Cleveland's side. Ball's righteous account was extravagantly exaggerated. He accused Cleveland of abusing Maria and neglecting the child. Grover's Buffalo apartment was, according to Ball, a "harem." The shocking story was reprinted in papers from coast to coast.

Cleveland's response to this bombshell was legendary: "Whatever you do," he wired his friends in Buffalo, "tell the truth." He admitted to the affair but denied abusing or neglecting either mother or child. His honesty won him more support than his indiscretion had cost him. "After the preliminary offense," one minister declared, "his conduct was singularly honorable." Cleveland's candor was commendable—and shrewd. He was already renowned as an ethical and hardworking governor who rooted out corruption and waste, and his handling of the Halpin affair cemented his reputation for honesty. He'd turned a potentially crippling scandal into a demonstration of integrity.

But the episode embittered Grover. He felt betrayed by his adopted hometown. When a friend invited him to Buffalo later that year, Grover declined. "I would never go there again if I could avoid it," he wrote.

The incident also instilled in him a fundamental hostility toward the press.

The 1884 presidential campaign still stands as one of the closest—and ugliest—ever. The candidates weren't very far apart on the issues, so the campaign devolved into mudslinging and character assassination. The Democrats called Blaine a liar and taunted him mercilessly with a chant:

> Blaine, Blaine, James G. Blaine
> The continental liar from the state of Maine

For their part, the Republicans portrayed Cleveland as a womanizing drunkard. Of course they also made much of the Halpin affair,

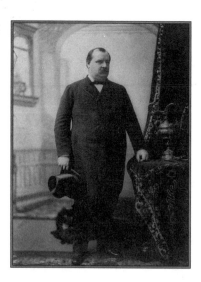

Grover Cleveland in 1888. Grover's weight would eventually approach three hundred pounds, making him quite literally the biggest political figure of his generation. LIBRARY OF CONGRESS

even commissioning a mocking song called "Ma! Ma! Where's My Pa?"

> Ma! Ma! Where is my pa?
> Up in the White House, darling
> Making the laws, working the cause
> Up in the White House, dear

Some of the bitterest attacks on Cleveland came from Charles Dana, the *New York Sun* editor whom Cleveland had alienated by refusing to hire his friend. Dana called Cleveland "a coarse debauchee who would bring his harlots with him to Washington and hire lodgings for them convenient to the White House." He also railed against Cleveland's "plodding mind, limited knowledge, and narrow capacities." It was Dana who sarcastically labeled Cleveland's reformist Republican supporters mugwumps, appropriating an old Algonquian word supposedly meaning "war leader." To Dana's consternation, the mugwumps embraced the label as a badge of honor.

The election came down to New York, the biggest electoral plum at the time. The candidate who won that state's thirty-six electoral votes would win the presidency. Since it was his home state, Cleveland should have had an advantage, but in the previous seven presidential elections the state had gone Democratic just twice: 1868 and 1876.

On October 29, 1884—just five days before the election—a Presbyterian minister introducing Blaine at an event in New York City condemned the Democrats as the party of "Rum, Romanism, and Rebellion"—drunk, Catholic, and disloyal. That single disparaging remark swung the Catholic vote in New York to Cleveland. That, coupled with the support of the mugwumps, helped Cleveland carry the state by 1,047 votes—out of 1.1 million cast. Nationwide, Cleveland won the popular vote by just 0.7 percent.

The margin was razor thin, but Grover Cleveland had ended the Republican Party's stranglehold on the White House. Jubilant Democrats came up with a new chant:

Hurrah for Maria
Hurrah for the kid
We voted for Grover
And we're damn glad we did

On March 4, 1885, Stephen Grover Cleveland became the first Democrat to assume the presidency in twenty-eight years. He also became just the second bachelor president, after James Buchanan. The first time he had ever stepped foot in Washington was the day before.

3

THE DREAD DISEASE

O N JUNE 2, 1884, at his summer home in Long Branch, New Jersey, Ulysses S. Grant bit into a peach and suddenly felt a sharp pain in his throat, a pain so intense it made him cry out. The retired general and former president, who had survived close calls in two wars, was nearly felled by a piece of fruit. As the summer progressed, the pain became more acute, especially when Grant swallowed, but it wasn't until November that Grant, by then having returned to his home in New York City, finally consented to an examination. He went to see Dr. John Hancock Douglas, who was one of the country's leading throat specialists. Douglas detected a small, scaly growth at the base of Grant's tongue.

"Is it cancer?" Grant bluntly asked the doctor.

"General," Douglas answered, "the disease is serious, epithelial in character, and sometimes capable of being cured."

In other words, yes.

Today, Grant would be diagnosed with a squamous cell carcinoma—the same type of cancer that Grover Cleveland would be diagnosed with nine years later.

In the nineteenth century, no diagnosis was as feared as cancer. It was tantamount to a death sentence. The very word was not spoken in polite company. It was most commonly referred to as "the dread disease" or simply "the disease." Even Dr. Douglas admitted he "avoided the use of the word 'cancer'" in front of Grant.

The phobia was well founded. Cancer had confounded doctors since the fifth century BC, when Hippocrates advised, "It is better not to apply treatment in cases of occult [internal] cancer; for if treated, the patients die quickly; but if not treated, they hold out for a long time." Indeed, the treatments were as fearsome, and nearly as fatal, as the disease. A Viennese doctor named Theodor Billroth was one of the nineteenth century's most skilled surgeons. He operated on 170 cancer patients between 1867 and 1876. Eight survived longer than three years—a survival rate of 4.7 percent. Inevitably, alternative remedies flourished. One of the most successful patent medicine peddlers in the United States was John D. Rockefeller's father, William Rockefeller, whose calling card claimed he could cure "all cases of cancer." He sold a liquid potion for twenty-five dollars a bottle. Folk remedies abounded as well. One called for the hand of a dead man to be placed on the tumor. Another prescribed the head of a puppy, dried and powdered and mixed with honey, to be applied to the growth.

Truth was, nobody knew what caused cancer or how to cure it. Some doctors believed it was contagious or hereditary. Others blamed luxurious living, melancholy blood, grief, anxiety, too much nourishing food, and very hot food or drink. In 1881, when a Boston medical journal offered a $1,000 prize for the best essay on the "Cure for a Malignant Disease," it received exactly three entries. When the journal reprised the contest a year later, it received none. The journal blamed the "barrenness of American researchers." Cancerphobia effectively stymied research. Medical schools and hospitals did not want to be associated with the disease. The first cancer hospital in the United States didn't open until 1905 in Philadelphia. Today it's known as the Fox Chase Cancer Center, but then it was called the American Oncologic Hospital, the word "cancer" being deemed still too alarming.

Of cancer, the Philadelphia surgeon Samuel Gross glumly declared in the middle of the nineteenth century, "all we know, with any degree of certainty, is that we know nothing."

Some theories, however, were beginning to emerge. An eighteenth-century English doctor named Percivall Pott noticed that chimney sweeps seemed to get cancer of the scrotum in unusually high numbers. He blamed soot. In the mid-nineteenth century, cancers of the mouth and throat became more common. Some doctors attributed it to the increased use of cigars and chewing tobacco. Grant was a heavy smoker—he was known to consume as many as twenty cigars a day—and his doctor, John Hancock Douglas, believed that "smoking was the exciting cause" of Grant's cancer. Still, the opinion was not universally shared. Grant's dentist, Frank Abbott, believed the "constant irritation" from the "rough and ragged surfaces of a broken tooth" had caused the cancer in Grant's mouth. "Tobacco probably had little or nothing to do with the origin of the tumor," Abbott said.

Much like AIDS a century later, the stigma attached to cancer was so deep and profound that people who had it were embarrassed or afraid to admit it, and Grant was no exception. He told no one outside his immediate family he had cancer. Even his closest friends were kept in the dark as to the true nature of his illness. When rumors about the general's health began to circulate in January 1885, his physicians flatly denied Grant had cancer, instead blaming his poor health on "a bothersome tooth." "Gen. Grant has not cancer of the tongue," Dr. Douglas fibbed to reporters. "The difficulty is in his mouth, and it is of an epithelial character. The irritation has now been greatly relieved, and that is all I feel at liberty to say." By then, however, Grant's doctors already knew he had a "cancer of the malignant type that was sure to end fatally." Surgery was deemed too risky. The cancer was too far advanced. By April it had spread to Grant's throat, neck, and soft palate. There was nothing Grant's doctors could do but try to ease his pain.

This they did with frequent doses of cocaine. Grant was grateful for the relief, however temporary. "I have tried to study the function of the use of cocain[e]," he wrote. "The conclusion I have come to in my case is, taken properly, it gives a wonderful amount of relief from pain."

As the disease progressed, it became impossible for Grant and his doctors to conceal the fact that Grant had cancer. Newspapers began a morbid deathwatch outside Grant's townhouse on East Sixty-Sixth Street, near Central Park. Reporters rented a house nearby and worked in shifts around the clock. Grant received a stream of well-wishers, each of whom was ambushed by reporters eager for some tidbit of information. Generally the newspaper reports were more fanciful than factual, and, in keeping with the journalistic standards of the day, many were total fabrications. One of the less credible reports claimed that in the middle of one night the general shouted out, "I can't stand it! I'm going to die!"

As he sank closer to death, Grant's illness was covered with a fervor verging on hysteria, with vivid reports detailing each "violent and alarming fit of coughing" in clinical detail. Never before had a famous American's battle with cancer been so thoroughly documented. It was the nineteenth-century equivalent of wall-to-wall coverage. A few of the bolder newspapers even used the word "cancer" itself.

The intense coverage of Grant's cancer did nothing to alleviate the public's fear of the disease. In fact, it only confirmed what was already widely believed: cancer was a killer that could not be stopped, "an alien and living invader." Or, as the *New York Tribune* put it, "a genuine case of malignant cancer is incurable."

General Grant's death was agonizing. The tumor slowly enlarged, making it impossible for him to swallow, to eat, and, eventually, to breathe. His body withered away. He lost a hundred pounds, nearly half his healthy weight. By June he was unable to speak and could only communicate by handwriting. He scrawled messages in pencil on brown slips of paper, many of which survive. Some of the notes are poignant. "I should prefer going now to enduring my present suffering for a single day without hope of recovery," says one. "I think I am a verb instead of a personal pronoun," says another. "A verb is anything that signifies to be; to do; or to suffer; I signify all three."

All the while, as he slowly suffocated, Grant raced furiously to complete his memoirs. In May 1884—the month before he bit into that peach—Grant had been swindled out of his life savings by a Wall Street con artist. To provide for his family after he was gone, Grant had agreed to sell the rights to his memoirs to Mark Twain. On the afternoon of July 19, 1885, Grant finished writing.* A few hours later, he wrote a letter to Dr. Douglas. "There is nothing more I should do to it now," he wrote, referring to his memoirs, "and therefore I am not likely to be more ready to go than at this moment."

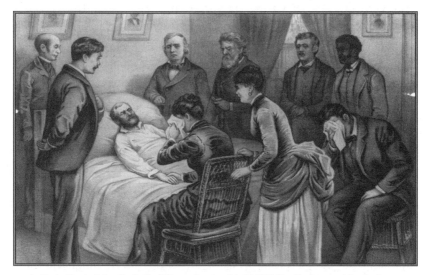

An illustration depicting the death of Ulysses Grant on July 23, 1885. Grant's slow, agonizing death from cancer was exhaustively covered by newspapers. Never before had a famous American's battle with the disease been so thoroughly documented. LIBRARY OF CONGRESS

Less than four days later, on the morning of July 23, he died in his bed surrounded by his family and his doctors. "There was no expiring sigh," Dr. Douglas remembered. "Life passed away so quietly, so peacefully, that, to be sure it had terminated, we waited a minute."

---

* Grant's two-volume set of memoirs would sell three hundred thousand copies and earn his survivors $500,000.

Grover Cleveland, who had begun his first term less than five months earlier, issued a proclamation. "The entire country has witnessed with deep emotion his prolonged and patient struggle with painful disease," Cleveland wrote, "and has watched by his couch of suffering with tearful sympathy."

Grant's funeral on August 8 in New York was one of the most spectacular outpourings of grief in history. An estimated 1.5 million people watched the seven-mile-long cortege slowly make its way from City Hall, up Broadway and Fifth Avenue, to Riverside Park. Black bunting hung from nearly every building along the route. General Winfield Scott Hancock, the hero of Gettysburg, led the procession, which lasted seven hours and included some sixty thousand marchers, including thousands of Civil War veterans. Men climbed telegraph poles just to catch a glimpse of Grant's catafalque as it passed. As Grant had wished, it was a reconciliatory event. Among the pallbearers were two Union generals and two Confederate generals. "I am sorry General Grant is dead," said Simon Bolivar Buckner, one of the Confederate pallbearers, "but his death has yet been the greatest blessing the country has ever received; now, reunion is perfect."

The catafalque was drawn by twenty-four black horses. Cleveland followed in a carriage pulled by six horses. Befitting the solemn occasion, Cleveland sat stone-faced, refusing to acknowledge the cheers that went up as he passed the teeming throngs.

When he emerged from his carriage for the interment at Riverside Park, it was obvious that Cleveland was not well. The "killing hours" he had kept as governor and, now, as president had plainly taken a toll on him. He had put on even more weight, and he walked with a pronounced limp, favoring his right leg, which was affected by gout.

But overwork alone was not to blame for Cleveland's poor health. Gout is a form of rheumatism that is caused by high levels of uric acid in the blood. The acid crystallizes in joints, often in the feet, causing severe pain. In Grover's day it was known as the rich man's disease, because it could be brought on by excessive consumption of meat, fish, and alcohol (especially beer) and aggravated by obesity. In cartoons, sufferers were caricatured as rich, fat, and lazy, sitting with bandaged feet resting on stools. Grover was certainly not lazy, but his gluttonous proclivities and aversion to exercise were practically a recipe for gout, and the ailment would plague him for the rest of his life.

But Cleveland found his bad habits impossible to break. When he'd moved into the White House, the new president had soon discovered he had no taste for the Gallic cuisine prepared by the White House chef, a Frenchman. "I must go to dinner," he wrote a friend. "I wish it was to eat a pickled herring, Swiss cheese and a chop at Louis' instead of the French stuff I shall find." One night Cleveland caught a whiff of something familiar outside his window as he sat down to dinner. He summoned William Sinclair, the White House steward.

"William, what is that smell?" the president asked.

"I am very sorry, sir, but that is the smell of the servants' dinner."

"What is it—corned beef and cabbage?"

"Yes."

"Well, William, take this dinner down to the servants and bring their dinner to me."

Cleveland pronounced it the best meal he'd had in months.

Cleveland eventually replaced the Frenchman with a woman named Eliza, who had been his cook at the governor's mansion in Albany. From then on his usual breakfast consisted of oatmeal, beefsteak, eggs or a chop, and coffee. Not exactly a light, well-balanced meal.

He also continued to smoke and drink. In the summer of 1885, Grover went hunting in the Adirondacks with some friends. Afterward, a hiker who passed the presidential party's campsite was taken aback by the large number of empty bottles left behind—and only some of them were water bottles. Two years later, during a tour of the South, Grover arrived at the Atlanta home of Senator Alfred Colquitt after a grueling day of travel in pouring rain. "Senator," said the dripping-wet president, "I must have a drink right away." But Colquitt was a committed prohibitionist. "There hadn't been a drop of liquor in the house since I lived in it," he recalled. The flustered senator hurriedly fetched a bottle of bourbon from a neighbor, and the president had his drink—reportedly the only drink that Colquitt ever served in his life.

—————⟆•••⟆—————

As president, Cleveland wielded his veto pen as ruthlessly as he had as mayor and governor. In his first term he vetoed an astounding 414 bills, twice as many as all his predecessors combined. Many of the bills were private pension bills for Civil War veterans. One bill would have given drought-stricken Texas farmers $10,000 to purchase seed grain. "Federal aid in such cases encourages the expectation of paternal care on the part of the government and weakens the sturdiness of our national character," he wrote in his veto message, "while it prevents the indulgence among our people of that kindly sentiment and conduct which strengthens the bonds of a common brotherhood." He would veto another 170 bills in his second term, for a total of 584 vetoes, second only to Franklin Roosevelt's 635 (and FDR served more than three terms). Cleveland generally took a hands-off approach to the presidency. He believed his foremost responsibility was to prevent the enactment of bad laws.

The highlight of his first term wasn't political, however; it was personal. A month after taking office, Grover invited Oscar Folsom's widow, Emma, and her daughter, Frances, to visit him in the White House. Several more visits from the Folsoms followed, and it was widely rumored that Grover and Emma were considering marriage. But the true object of Grover's affection was Frances. "I don't see why the papers keep marrying me to old ladies all the while," the president quipped.

Grover and Frances were an odd couple: He was burly and gruff. She was petite and charming. And, of course, there was the age difference—Grover was twenty-eight years older than Frances. He had practically been her guardian after her father was killed in a carriage accident. He had bought her a puppy when she was a little girl, and she'd called him Uncle Cleve. But as Frances matured, their feelings for each other blossomed into romance. When Frances went off to college at Wells, Grover sent her flowers regularly, and they corresponded faithfully. Grover was determined to hide their fledgling relationship from the papers, however. The lovebirds were never seen in public. When Frances visited the White House, she and Grover would spend evenings walking around the mansion and chatting. "Poor girl," Grover would say to her years later, "you never had any courting like other girls."

Grover proposed to Frances by letter in August 1885, shortly before she and her mother embarked on a nine-month European vacation to celebrate Frances's graduation from Wells. Frances accepted Grover's proposal by return post. The wedding took place in the Blue Room of the White House on the evening of June 2, 1886, just six days after Frances returned from Europe. It was an intimate ceremony: just twenty-eight guests, including all the members of the cabinet and their wives, excepting Attorney General Augustus Garland, who, after the death of his wife several years earlier, had pledged to never again take part in "social festivities," declining even to attend his own son's wedding. The forty-nine-year-old groom donned a tuxedo with a white bowtie. The twenty-one-year-old bride wore a gown of heavy corded satin so stiff it could stand up by itself. Grover's brother William, a Presbyterian minister, presided. In her vows, Frances promised to "love, honor, and . . . keep"—not "obey." The music was provided by the Marine Band under the direction of John Philip Sousa.

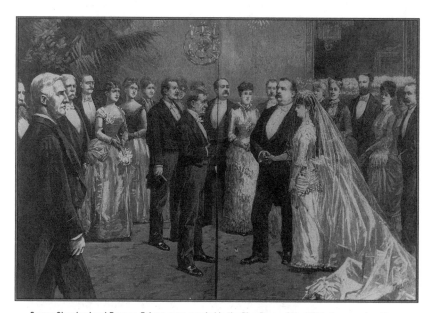

Grover Cleveland and Frances Folsom were married in the Blue Room of the White House on June 2, 1886. Cleveland is the only president to have been married in the mansion. He would not allow the ceremony to be photographed. LIBRARY OF CONGRESS

Frances Cleveland became the youngest First Lady in history and one of the most beloved. William H. Crook, a longtime White House employee, remembered her arrival on the morning of the wedding. "She tripped up the steps, and swept through the great entrance like a radiant vision of young springtime . . . from that instant every man and woman of them all was a devoted slave, and remained such." Pretty, witty, and unaffected, Frances proved to be an exceptional hostess, and she became Grover's greatest political asset. One of his political enemies once declared, "I detest him so much that I don't even think his wife is beautiful."

The Clevelands honeymooned at Deer Park, a resort in the mountains of western Maryland. They were followed by hordes of reporters, some of whom camped outside their simple rented cottage, peering through the windows and following the couple on their strolls through the woods. Their every move was described in detail for millions of delighted readers. Naturally, this circus did not improve Grover's opinion of reporters in general.

In fact, his relationship with the press only deteriorated as his presidency progressed. Of course, this was partly because reporters incessantly hounded him and Frances. But it was also a product of Grover's personality. He was almost pathologically reserved, practically Nixonian in his social awkwardness. As a result, he was bewildered, frustrated, and outraged by the inordinate attention the papers paid to his personal life, and sometimes he was unable to contain his fury. In 1885 he fired off a letter to the publisher of the popular magazine *Puck*. "The falsehoods daily spread before the people in our newspapers," he wrote, "are insults to the American love for decency and fair play of which we boast." In a letter to the *New York Evening Post*, he condemned "keyhole correspondents." "They have used the enormous power of the modern newspaper to perpetuate and disseminate a colossal impertinence, and have done it, not as professional gossips and tattlers, but as the guides and instructors of the public in conduct and morals."

Without the benefit of a bona fide press secretary, Cleveland was largely left to his own devices when it came to dealing with the press. On a vacation to the Adirondacks he considered selecting one reporter to accompany him and send reports to all the papers wishing to receive them—perhaps the earliest attempt at pool reporting. But, for the most part, he was helpless in the face of the braying papers. In 1886, Cleveland was giving a speech at Harvard when he noticed a group of reporters sitting at a table near the podium. "At once his voice and posture changed," Harvard president Charles Eliot later recalled. "He uttered several denunciatory sentences on the conduct of the press towards himself as a man and towards the President of the United States; and . . . tears rolled down his cheeks . . . tears of wrath and indignation."

Cleveland's fulmination, however, was selective. He was too shrewd to alienate indiscriminately. He realized he needed some allies in the newspaper business, and he counted a handful of prominent editors among his friends. But in general, he had no use for newspaper reporters. "Ghouls" he once called them. And when the time came, he would have no reservations about lying to them.

In 1888, Cleveland ran for reelection. His opponent this time was Benjamin Harrison, a bearded and humorless Civil War general and former senator from Indiana. In stark contrast to the previous campaign, this one, in the words of one political reporter, was "conducted on both sides with . . . dignity and decency."

It was another nail-biter. Once again the election came down to New York, but this time Cleveland could not carry the state, losing by less than 1 percent of the vote. Despite losing the electoral vote, Cleveland still managed to win the popular vote (a scenario that would not be repeated until 2000). When Frances Cleveland moved out of the White House on March 4, 1889, she told a servant named Jerry Smith, "Now, Jerry, I want you to take care of all the furniture and ornaments in the house, for I want to find everything just as it is now when we come back again."

Smith gasped in disbelief.

"We are coming back just four years from today," Frances predicted.

The Clevelands retreated to a handsome brownstone at 816 Madison Avenue in New York City. Grover practiced a bit of law, mostly acting as an arbitrator in business disputes. The couple didn't go out much. They primarily socialized with a small but influential circle of friends, including actor Joseph Jefferson, banker Elias C. Benedict, and journalists L. Clarke Davis and Richard Watson Gilder. It was certainly a more highfalutin crowd than Grover had hung with when he was a bachelor in Buffalo. Now he was consorting with what one acquaintance described as "a millionaire's crowd." There would be no more German beer gardens with sawdust-covered floors. In New York, he was much closer to Wall Street, both literally and figuratively. He grew more sympathetic to the needs of bankers and business owners and less sensitive to the concerns of ordinary workers like his erstwhile friends in the saloons along Canal Street in Buffalo.

A few minutes after midnight on October 3, 1891, Frances and Grover's first child was born at the brownstone on Madison Avenue. Her name was Ruth, and her birth was front-page news. The papers dubbed her Baby Ruth and shamelessly reported her infantile exploits as news: "Baby Ruth . . . shook her chubby little hand to the crowd about the car window" (*New York Tribune*, September 1, 1893). Ruth was as beloved as her mother. In 1890, the year before her birth, the name Ruth had been the forty-sixth most popular for girls born in the United States. In 1892, it was fifth.

The Clevelands' eldest child, it is worth noting here, has long been cited as the eponym for the Baby Ruth candy bar, but the evidence is unconvincing. Ruth would die of diphtheria in 1904. The candy bar debuted in 1921—just as the baseball slugger Babe Ruth was emerging as a national idol. By insisting that the bar was named for the dead daughter of a dead president, the Curtiss Candy Company successfully avoided compensating the home run king. Even Nestlé, the company that makes the bar today, acknowledges that "many theories surround the origin of the Baby Ruth name."

Buoyed by sweeping Democratic victories in the midterm elections of 1890, Cleveland began dabbling in national politics once again. The

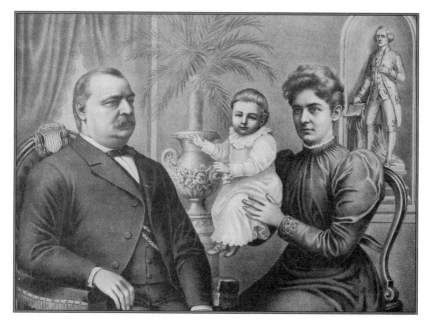

The Cleveland family in 1893: Grover, Ruth, and Frances. LIBRARY OF CONGRESS

passage of the Silver Purchase Act in July 1890 had made the money question more urgent than ever, and in February 1891, Cleveland made his position on the contentious issue perfectly clear. In an open letter, he called "the unlimited coinage of silver" a "dangerous and reckless experiment." By unequivocally aligning himself with the pro-gold, Eastern wing of the Democratic Party, Cleveland risked alienating pro-silver Democrats in the South and West. It was widely believed he had blown his chance to win the nomination in 1892, though he didn't seem to mind. "At any rate," he said, "no one can doubt where I stand." And he decided to seek the nomination anyway.

At the Democratic convention in Chicago in June 1892, Cleveland, as expected, faced fierce opposition from pro-silver delegates, as well as his old nemesis Tammany Hall. But he still won the nomination on the first ballot, mainly because he was the only candidate with a realistic chance of actually winning the election. The silverites, however, won a consolation prize: Cleveland's running mate would be former Illinois congressman Adlai Stevenson, whose stance on the money question was precisely the opposite of Cleveland's. Stevenson favored the free coinage of silver. Cleveland wasn't happy, but it was hardly an unusual situation. Presidential candidates did not begin choosing their own running mates until the 1940s. Before then, the vice presidential nominee was chosen at the party's convention—usually with little input from the man at the top of the ticket. This inevitably led to some uncomfortable arranged marriages. Garfield and Arthur, for instance, were barely on speaking terms. It was, however, highly unusual for a president and vice president to be on opposite sides of the most fractious political issue of the day, as were Cleveland and Stevenson on the money question.

Stevenson's nomination balanced the ticket and mollified the silverites somewhat, but it would come back to haunt Cleveland.

The 1892 campaign was even more tranquil than the campaign four years earlier had been. According to one historian, it was "the cleanest, quietest, and most creditable" since the Civil War. Truth was, the candidates hardly campaigned at all. Benjamin Harrison's wife, Caroline, had contracted tuberculosis, and Harrison barely left her side. Cleveland refused to campaign as well, citing what he called the "afflictive dispensation of Providence."*

Mostly Cleveland whiled away the 1892 campaign at Gray Gables, his summer home on Cape Cod, fishing in Buzzards Bay and nursing his gout. Caroline Harrison died in the White House on October 25. Exactly two weeks later, Cleveland trounced Harrison in the most lopsided presidential election since Lincoln's second victory in 1864. Cleveland carried twenty-three states, Harrison sixteen. James B. Weaver, the candidate of the pro-silver Populist Party, won four states. Cleveland won the popular vote by 3 percent, and he is still the only president besides FDR to have won the popular vote in more than two elections. The Democrats also captured both houses of Congress.

---

* This was a typically Clevelandian turn of phrase. "He had a tendency to mount polysyllabic stilts," one of his secretaries recalled.

Harrison's undoing was the federal budget. He was the first president to sign a billion-dollar budget, and the Democrats made government spending a campaign issue. Not that Harrison minded losing. In fact, he seemed relieved. "For me there is no sting in it," he said. "Indeed after the heavy blow the death of my wife dealt me, I do not think I could have stood the strain a reelection would have brought."

On March 4, 1893, the Clevelands returned to the White House, exactly as Frances had predicted four years earlier. As she'd requested, everything was just as the Clevelands had left it, with one notable exception: the Harrisons had replaced the gas lights with electric lights.

Less than four months later, on the morning of Friday, June 23, Dr. Joseph Bryant examined the rough spot on the roof of Grover's mouth and pronounced it a "bad looking tenant" that should be evicted post-haste. Fortunately, Bryant said, the tumor had been detected early. It could be removed surgically, though, as Bryant well knew, the procedure would be risky. Just three years earlier, Bryant had authored a paper on the removal of oral tumors. He reported a mortality rate of 14 percent.

That afternoon, Bryant and White House physician Robert O'Reilly consulted with the president in his office above the East Room. Joining them was Dan Lamont, Cleveland's close friend and former private secretary, who was now his secretary of war. The four men discussed, as Bryant later wrote, "the final removal of the disease, and the time and place of the operative procedure." The tone was grave. Grover, sitting behind his massive *Resolute* desk, stroked his moustache compulsively, as was his habit when deep in thought. The discussion lasted into the evening, and the men made decisions that had the potential to alter the course of American history.

The first decision: keep everything secret. "During the discussion," Bryant recalled, "the president would not under any circumstances consent to the operative removal of the disease at a time or place that would not give the best opportunity of avoiding disclosures and even a suspicion that anything of significance had happened to him." But

there was a catch: secrecy was possible only if the surgery left no visible
scars. It was possible, Bryant assured Cleveland, to perform the operation entirely within Cleveland's mouth, without an external incision.
But only if the cancer had not spread too far.

Cleveland had two reasons for keeping his cancer secret. The first
was political. If it came to be known he had the dread disease, he
believed public confidence in the economy, already badly shaken, would
be utterly shattered. Republican Wall Street, always suspicious of the
Democratic president, would abandon him. The silverites would seize
the opportunity to save the Silver Purchase Act. And, in the words of
Dr. Bryant, the panic would "become a rout." Cleveland was not being
vain. It was widely believed that his health and the nation's health were
inextricably linked. In an editorial published before the full extent of
his illness was even known, the *Commercial and Financial Chronicle* wrote,
"Mr. Cleveland is about all that stands between this country and absolute disaster, and his death would be a great calamity." Apart from Dan
Lamont, not even his cabinet was to know. Cleveland was especially adamant that the truth be concealed from Adlai Stevenson, his pro-silver
vice president. Cleveland's failure to inform even his potential successor
of the operation was uncharacteristically reckless. If the president died
in surgery or was otherwise disabled, Stevenson would be wholly unpre-
pared to assume power.[*]

The second reason for secrecy was personal. As mentioned, Cleveland was by nature intensely private. He had witnessed firsthand the
ghoulish hoopla surrounding Ulysses Grant's illness, and he had no
intention of becoming the object of such a spectacle. Cleveland, Bryant
wrote, had a "strong desire to avoid the notoriety naturally incident to
public knowledge" of his illness.

The four men then discussed the timing of the operation. Bryant
wanted it to take place immediately, but Cleveland said he needed some

---

[*] In 1967, seventy-four years after Cleveland's operation, the Twenty-Fifth Amendment was
ratified. It provides for the temporary transfer of power to the vice president when a president is
incapacitated.

time to get things in order first. "I cannot leave here before the end of the month [June] under any circumstances," the president said. "Therefore, since the time must be set, I will say to you that I will be ready on the first day of July." And so it was decided that the operation would take place on Saturday, July 1.

Finally, there was the crucial matter of place. It was quickly concluded that it would be impossible for the operation to be performed in a hospital. The risk of leaks was far too great. Gray Gables, the president's summer home on Buzzards Bay, was briefly considered but also rejected—too many reporters snooping around. At Cleveland's suggestion, it was ultimately decided that the best place for the operation would be the *Oneida*, a luxury yacht owned by the tycoon "Commodore" Elias Benedict, who was a close friend of the president. (Benedict was no more a commodore than Dan Lamont was a colonel.) Cleveland had logged more than fifty thousand miles on the *Oneida*, mostly fishing in Long Island Sound and off the coast of Cape Cod. His presence on the boat would arouse no suspicions whatsoever. The surgical team and equipment would be boarded surreptitiously before the president. The operation would take place while the boat sailed from New York to Gray Gables. For all the world it would look like the president was simply sailing to his summer home for a well-deserved respite. It was a simple solution, though the doctors understood it would pose some unusual and potentially dangerous problems.

Unspoken was the very real possibility that Cleveland would suffer the same fate as General Grant. If the tumor had grown too large to remove, the president, like the general, would meet a most unpleasant demise, slowly suffocating.

It was agreed that Bryant would return to New York to assemble the surgical team. Lamont would assist with the preparations from Washington. O'Reilly would monitor the patient until the operation.

President Cleveland, meanwhile, had one week to ponder his fate— and the nation's—before the operation.

The four men must have shared a good stiff drink before adjourning for the night.

Grover Cleveland was not the first president to attempt to conceal an illness from the public, and he would certainly not be the last. George Washington tried to hide the fact that he contracted influenza during his first term. The illness—which nearly killed him—left the nation leaderless for several weeks. In November 1863, shortly after delivering the Gettysburg Address, Abraham Lincoln came down with smallpox, which his aides dismissed as "varioloid," the mildest form of the disease. In fact, Lincoln had the most virulent form of smallpox, and it took him more than a month to recover—at one of the most crucial moments in the nation's history. When the Associated Press reported that President Chester Arthur was suffering from a fatal kidney ailment called Bright's disease in 1882, Arthur categorically denied the report, but less than two years after leaving office, he died of complications from the disease.*

Loath to appear weak in any way, some presidents have gone to remarkable lengths to hide their infirmities. On October 2, 1919, shortly after returning to the White House from a grueling nationwide speaking tour, Woodrow Wilson suffered a massive stroke. What followed was a most audacious cover-up. The stroke paralyzed the left side of Wilson's body and incapacitated him so completely, physically and mentally, that, in the words of historian Robert Ferrell, "The president should have resigned immediately." Instead, the White House physician, Cary T. Grayson, announced that Wilson was merely suffering from "nervous exhaustion." For four months Wilson conducted virtually no official business, and for the remaining thirteen months of his term, Ferrell writes, "he could hardly focus his mind on any piece of public business beyond, say, ten minutes or so, after which he tired." It was another critical moment in our history: At the time, the Senate was debating ratification of the Treaty of Versailles, which ended World

---

* Arthur, apparently aware of his imminent demise, campaigned only halfheartedly for the Republican nomination in 1884. This, coupled with Arthur's reformist tendencies, resulted in the nomination of James G. Blaine, who ultimately lost the election to Cleveland.

War I and created the League of Nations. Without Wilson's leadership, the treaty was doomed. The Senate rejected it by a vote of fifty-three to thirty-eight.

Wilson had suffered his first stroke in 1896 at age thirty-nine. Two more followed, in 1904 and 1906. The electorate knew nothing of Wilson's health problems, however. The square-jawed son of a Presbyterian minister, Wilson projected an image of stern vigor, and he was elected governor of New Jersey in 1910 and president of the United States in 1912 and 1916, making him the first Democrat to capture the White House since Grover Cleveland in 1892.

Like Cleveland, Wilson concealed his ailment even from his own cabinet. For four months after the stroke, only his doctors, his private secretary, and his wife, Edith, were permitted to see him. What little business that was transacted went through Edith, whom Wilson had married in 1915, a little more than a year after the death of his first wife. Papers sent to the president were returned with notes in Mrs. Wilson's handwriting, not the president's. Edith Wilson, for all intents and purposes, oversaw the executive branch after her husband's stroke. It has been said that she could be considered the country's first female president.

Also like Cleveland, Wilson was especially eager to hide the truth from his would-be successor. After the stroke, Vice President Thomas Marshall didn't see Wilson until the day the two men left office.

It wasn't until February 10, 1920—more than four months after the stroke—that one of Wilson's doctors finally admitted to a *Baltimore Sun* reporter that the president had, in fact, suffered a "cerebral thrombosis." By then, of course, it was obvious that something was gravely amiss. Wilson, now a recluse with a white beard, hadn't been seen in public since the stroke. Still, the White House continued the charade that the president was well. In April 1920, a clean-shaven Wilson finally reconvened his cabinet. At meetings he sat propped up in a chair, White House usher Ike Hoover remembered, "as one in a trance." Wilson said almost nothing at the meetings. What little he did say was barely intelligible. After the first cabinet meeting "dragged on for more than an hour," Mrs. Wilson stepped in to stop it. "The stories in the papers from day to day may have been true in their way," Hoover said, "but never was deception so universally practiced in the White House as it was in those statements being given out from time to time."

Wilson's term ended on March 4, 1921. Despite pressing domestic problems, including rampant inflation and widespread racial and labor strife, Wilson accomplished nothing after the stroke. He never fully recovered, and he died less than three years after leaving office.

Presidents have not always received the best health care available, often because they've chosen their health care providers poorly. Like so many other appointments, a president's choice of White House physician is often based on sentiment or politics, not on expertise. Wilson's White House physician, Cary Grayson, lucked into the job. Grayson, who attended medical school for just one year, happened to attend a luncheon at the White House shortly after Wilson's inauguration. During the luncheon, Wilson's sister tripped and cut her forehead. Grayson stitched the wound, winning Wilson's gratitude—and a plum job. (It helped that Grayson, like Wilson, was a native Virginian.) Another doctor might not have allowed the frail president to undertake the speaking tour that immediately preceded his stroke.

Wilson's successor, Warren Harding, was a genial nincompoop who chose as his White House physician the hopelessly unqualified Charles Sawyer, an old family friend and archetypal small-town doctor. Sawyer practiced homeopathy, a form of alternative medicine in which patients are prescribed tiny doses of substances that replicate the very symptoms that are meant to be cured. For example, a patient with insomnia might be prescribed a tall glass of water with a few drops of coffee. The underpinning theory articulated by Samuel Hahnemann, the German doctor who invented homeopathy more than two hundred years ago, is that like cures like. Homeopathy had been widely discredited by the time Harding became president, but Dr. Sawyer was not persuaded. Sawyer was also fond of prescribing pills by color. Once he prescribed the president a dose of soda water and two pink pills.

When he became president, Harding's systolic pressure was 180 (it should have been 140 or less). His heart was so weak that it was unable to pump blood out of his lungs. As a result, Harding had to sleep propped up with pillows. If he slept lying down, blood would pool in his lungs, making it difficult for him to breathe. Even his valet knew Harding was deathly ill, telling a Secret Service agent that "something is going to happen to our boss." A better doctor certainly would have noticed the unmistakable symptoms of heart disease, but Sawyer didn't.

In the summer of 1923, Harding undertook a punishing tour of Alaska and the West Coast. The heat was scorching, and the president weakened by the day. He could barely stand. His speech was slurred. On the night of July 27, Harding went to bed in Seattle complaining of painful cramps. He had probably suffered a heart attack, but Sawyer dismissed it as a touch of food poisoning. Six days later, in Room 8064 of the Palace Hotel in San Francisco, Harding's heart stopped beating. Officially, the cause of death was ruled a stroke, though the underlying cause was undoubtedly congestive heart failure.

But when it comes to presidents receiving bad health care, it's hard to top poor old James Garfield. As if getting shot twice by Charles Guiteau at a Washington train station on July 2, 1881, wasn't bad enough, Garfield was then subjected to some real Keystone Kops doctoring. One of the bullets harmlessly grazed his right arm, but the other entered his lower back. The first doctor on the scene stuck his dirty finger into the wound in Garfield's back to determine the path of the bullet and, if possible, remove it. The second doctor on the scene did the same thing. The president was taken back to the White House. X-rays were still unknown at the time, and over the next twenty-four hours more than a dozen doctors probed the president's wound with unwashed fingers and unsterilized instruments, futilely attempting to locate the bullet. This triggered an infection that could have been cured only with medicines yet undiscovered.

Outside Garfield's room, his doctors began to argue among themselves about the best course of treatment. Some advocated immediate surgery. Others argued the risk was too great. Tensions ran so high that a fistfight broke out. No surgery was performed.

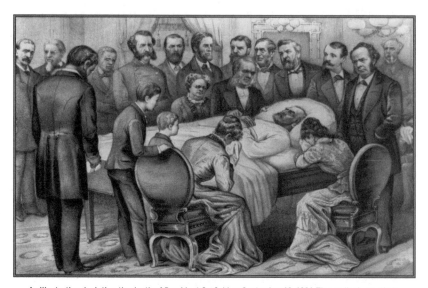

An illustration depicting the death of President Garfield on September 19, 1881. The medical care that Garfield received after he was shot was so shoddy that he probably would have been better off—and might have lived—if his doctors had never touched him. LIBRARY OF CONGRESS

Notably, Garfield's White House physician, Jedediah Baxter, was not among the doctors attending the wounded president. Baxter was an excellent physician, but, due to a toxic combination of professional jealousy and personal animosity, the other doctors refused him access to Garfield.*

At one point, Garfield's doctors enlisted Alexander Graham Bell to help find the bullet lodged inside the president. Bell and another inventor named Simon Newcomb had devised a crude metal detector fashioned out of wire coils, a battery, and a telephone receiver. But when they passed the contraption over Garfield's body, it seemed to detect metal everywhere. The inventors were deeply disappointed by their failure. What they didn't realize was that the president was lying on a brand-new mattress with coil bedsprings, a recent innovation at the time.

---

* Given the dismal outcome, the snub probably saved Baxter's career. He would later serve as Benjamin Harrison's White House physician and surgeon general of the army.

Garfield's condition did not improve. The infection ravaged him. Pus oozed from his wound and filled his salivary glands, swelling his face. His weight dropped precipitously. He lingered until September 19.

If his doctors had never touched him, Garfield most likely would have survived. The bullet, it turned out, had lodged harmlessly in tissue. It hadn't killed Garfield; his doctors' obsession with finding it had. At his trial, Charles Guiteau argued—rather convincingly, according to many witnesses—that he was not responsible for Garfield's death: the president's doctors, by their incompetence, had killed him. It was compelling stuff, but the jury didn't buy it. Guiteau was hanged on June 30, 1882.

At least Grover Cleveland was in better hands. His personal physician, Joseph Bryant, was a former New York City health commissioner and an accomplished surgeon with a thriving practice said to be worth $25,000 a year (about $600,000 in today's money). He was also a professor of surgery at Bellevue Hospital Medical College, and he would go on to serve as president of the American Medical Association. Bryant was a friend of Dan Lamont—their wives were sisters—and it was Lamont who had introduced Bryant to Cleveland shortly after Cleveland was elected governor. Bryant and Cleveland hit it off immediately, and the two men frequently went hunting and fishing together.

Cleveland undoubtedly asked Bryant to be his White House physician, but Bryant was probably reluctant to abandon his lucrative private practice. So Cleveland turned to Robert O'Reilly, whose army biography describes him as having "great personal attraction, winning the affection and loyalty of all with whom he came into intimate contact." O'Reilly had served as a Union medic in the Civil War. After the war, he attended medical school at the University of Pennsylvania, graduating in 1866. He returned to the army, and, after a stint fighting the Sioux in Wyoming, he was assigned to Washington, where "his attractive personality and his professional skill made him a prominent figure in the capital." Apparently O'Reilly was a charming raconteur and accomplished violinist who killed at parties. Shortly after Cleveland arrived in

Washington, he struck up an "intimate and agreeable" friendship with O'Reilly and appointed him White House physician. O'Reilly was a capable doctor, and he would go on to become chairman of the American Red Cross.

But even having the best doctors doesn't guarantee the best care, especially when the patient is a president. Proximity to power can cloud judgment. "The success of the presidential patient's political agenda becomes intertwined with the success of the physician," writes medical historian Ludwig Deppisch. "As a result, secrecy and misdirection can exaggerate and distort the traditional . . . doctor-patient relationship." That was certainly the case with Grover Cleveland. By insisting on total secrecy, the president, not his doctors, dictated his course of treatment.

Ponder for a moment the decisions that were made in the White House that warm early summer evening in 1893. The president has a cancerous tumor in his mouth but consents to its removal only if the operation is performed on a friend's yacht and at a time of his choosing. The plan, Deppisch writes, "was hardly propitious for a successful conclusion."

Considering the risks, it's hard to believe Joseph Bryant and Robert O'Reilly ever agreed to perform the operation at all. That they did is a testament to their courage and patriotism—as well as their vanity and foolishness.

In the vernacular of their times, if anything went wrong, they'd be up to the hub in mud.

4

DR. KEEN

O N FRIDAY, JUNE 23, 1893, the same day that plans were first
hatched for the secret operation, Joseph Bryant sent a letter by
special delivery to his friend William Williams Keen, the head of surgery at Jefferson Medical College in Philadelphia. In the letter, Bryant
cryptically asked Keen to meet him as soon as possible to discuss "a very
important private matter." Keen was intrigued, and a little unnerved; he
was anxious to find out what merited such urgency—and such secrecy.
On the following Monday, Keen would be in New York to catch a ferry
to Providence. He immediately wired Bryant, suggesting they meet on
the deck of the ferry at 4:00 P.M. that day. The boat wasn't sailing until
6:15 that evening. It would be deserted. There they could discuss the
"private matter" undisturbed.

So, on June 26, Bryant met Keen on the empty ferry, which was
docked at Pier 28 on the North River, now better known as the Hudson. It was raining lightly. Bryant and Keen took seats in wooden deck
chairs. Each was impeccably dressed in a dark suit.

Bryant began by gravely announcing, "Mr. Cleveland is suffering from a serious disease of his upper left jaw." He went on to explain that an operation would be performed on the president in five days on board the *Oneida*, Commodore Elias Benedict's yacht. The whole matter was being kept secret—for the nation's sake, of course. Bryant said he was in the process of assembling a team of the finest surgeons for the operation, and he asked Keen if he would be willing to take part.

W. W. Keen was fifty-six years old and at the pinnacle of a long and exceedingly eminent career that practically spanned the chasm between medieval and modern medicine. He was the most celebrated surgeon in the nation. His reputation was unimpeachable. And now he was being asked to risk it all—for a president he hadn't even voted for.

William Williams Keen was born in 1837—the same year as Grover Cleveland. But there the similarities end, for Keen was everything the president was not: pious, sober, almost Puritanical. Their upbringings were vastly different, too. Keen's father had been a successful leather merchant in Philadelphia. The family had lived in a mansion—complete with a drawing room, chandeliers, and servants—at Thirty-Sixth and Chestnut Streets, in what was then the "country," where they raised corn and potatoes and even a cow and some chickens. On Sundays the

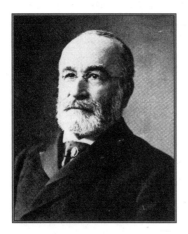

William Williams Keen was one of the country's most famous doctors when he was asked to join the surgical team that would secretly operate on the president. Keen's career spanned from the Civil War to World War I.
NATIONAL LIBRARY OF MEDICINE

family ate cold roast beef, "so as to give the cook as little work as possible on the Sabbath."

Keen's parents were strict Baptists, and a fear of God was instilled in Billy early. He was a serious young man, though he also enjoyed playing hockey and baseball. His later interest in medicine was probably sparked by his family's afflictions. He was the sixth of eight children, of whom only three survived childhood. Two of his siblings died of scarlet fever before he was born. Another died of diphtheria when Keen was twelve. When he was in his teens, his mother began falling regularly. "At first, we thought it was due to awkwardness and used to tease her about it in good humor," Keen remembered. "After a while we recognized the fact that her falls were due to a muscular weakness in her legs." Her arms were similarly affected. Perhaps she had ALS, also known as Lou Gehrig's disease. She would die in 1877, bedridden, paralyzed, and unable to feed herself.

Keen developed what he called a "love of order and exactness" at an early age. A good student, he was interested mostly in science, especially experimentation. As a young boy, he charted the growth of some grapevines in his backyard. One day he noted that a vine had grown one and three-quarter inches in just two hours. "Using a good magnifying glass, I could have literally *seen* it grow," he wrote many years later. "I have often been sorry that I did not repeat this kind of observation a number of times, to determine what the maximum rate of growth might be— and not only in grapes but also in other plants."

Keen was just sixteen when he graduated from Central High School, Philadelphia's most prestigious public school. He then spent two years studying with a private tutor before going to college at Brown. He later said he went to Brown for its progressive curriculum, which permitted students to choose their own courses, but he also chose it because it was a Baptist school. Keen planned to become a minister, though in college he would find a different calling.

Keen flowered at Brown. He joined a fraternity. Despite standing just five foot five, he played football and rowed. And he began dating. The object of his greatest affection was seventeen-year-old Emma Corinna

Borden (a second cousin of the infamous Lizzie Borden), who attended a finishing school in Providence. Tinnie, as she was known, was the daughter of one of the richest businessmen in Fall River, Massachusetts. Keen fell in love with Tinnie, but his love was not immediately requited.

At Brown, Keen also came under the spell of a charismatic and unorthodox science professor named George Ide Chace. Chace gave free lectures to Providence's metalworkers, dabbled in metaphysics, and frequently invited students to his home for supper. He was also a bit of a heretic; his more conservative colleagues found him "dangerously rationalistic." Keen, however, believed Chace was a "mastermind." He later wrote, "I could hardly wait from one recitation to the next." He especially enjoyed Chace's lectures on anatomy and biology.

Keen's enthusiasm for science tempered his passion for the pulpit. By his senior year he'd decided he wasn't suited for ministry. His religious convictions were changing. He no longer took the Bible literally and didn't believe in the virgin birth. He called this his "anxious period of doubt." He emerged from it "into a broader, happier, sunny belief in the goodness, mercy and love of God." Keen remained a devout Baptist for the rest of his life, but he came to detest religious fundamentalism.

Keen graduated from Brown at the top of his class in 1859—the same year Charles Darwin published *The Origin of Species*. The book had a profound effect on Keen, who was fascinated by what he called the "unfolding of human development." Keen was one of Darwin's earliest and most ardent advocates in North America and probably the first prominent American Baptist to publicly promote the theory of evolution. Keen had no difficulty reconciling science and religion. Evolution did not shake his faith. "To me," he wrote, "the Bible is the Book of Books. It is a precious manual of Religion but not a textbook of science."

Instead of entering the seminary, Keen had decided to enter medical school. Eager to return to Philadelphia, he applied for admission to Jefferson Medical College and was accepted. He moved back into his parents' house. He would live with them until he was almost thirty.

On the morning of Monday, October 8, 1860, Keen woke early and put on his best suit. He climbed into his landau and told his coachman to drive him downtown. The inside of the carriage smelled of mink oil, and the leather seats gleamed. The fastidious Keen liked his carriage to be kept clean. Slowly, steadily, the horses made their way over the Market Street Bridge to the heart of the city, their hooves clip-clopping on the cobblestone streets. Union Jacks festooned the lampposts, hung in honor of the Prince of Wales (later King Edward VII), who was coming to Philadelphia the very next day. He would be the first British royal to visit what was once the second largest city in the empire.

At Tenth and Sansom Streets, the carriage stopped in front of a saloon. Upstairs was Jefferson's infirmary, two dim rooms with five or six beds each. Keen, a confirmed teetotaler, must have smiled at the irony. The medical school itself was in a building across the street. Keen stepped out of the carriage and began his medical career.

There were sixty-five medical schools in the United States in 1860. None were regulated, licensed, or formally accredited. Few required even a high school diploma for admission. Most were operated solely for profit, with dreadful faculties and facilities. Things weren't much better fifty years later, when a Carnegie Foundation report on the state of medical education in the United States concluded that "there has been an enormous overproduction of uneducated and ill-trained medical practitioners."

Jefferson was better than that. Its admission standards were high and its faculty among the finest in the nation. The chairman of surgery was Samuel Gross, the most famous surgeon of his age. Gross was known as the Emperor of American Surgery, a title he wasn't inclined to refute.

But in 1860, even Jefferson—or Jeff, as it is sometimes called—was wanting. The school didn't even own a single microscope. The table that was used for cadaver dissections was also used for operations on living patients.

At the time, surgery was, in Keen's words, "crude and simple." Some doctors had begun experimenting with anesthetics, but they were not yet widely available. Keen remembered the first operation he witnessed at Jefferson as being rather gruesome. "I had just eaten my luncheon. By throwing out all my grappling hooks, I barely succeeded in holding it down." Before they performed operations, surgeons rarely bothered to wash their hands—much less their instruments—for they knew nothing of germs. In fact, most doctors stored their instruments in velvet-lined cases, a veritable breeding ground for bacteria. Surgeons worked in heavy black dress jackets covered with the blood of scores of operations. They wore the soiled jackets with pride, for the accumulation of crusty bloodstains attested to their surgical experience. Operating rooms were dark and filthy. Hospitals—of which there were fewer than two hundred in the nation—were considered places where people went to die, not to be made well. "The wards were full of fear," Keen remembered.

Just seventeen months after he entered Jefferson, Keen received his medical degree. It was March 1862, and Keen, a fervent abolitionist, offered his services to the Union Army. He was commissioned an acting assistant surgeon and spent much of the Civil War in hospitals, studying gunshot wounds, but on August 30, 1862, the last day of the Second Battle of Bull Run, he was unexpectedly ordered to Manassas. Keen led a convoy of thirty-six wagons from Washington to the battlefield. In Centreville, Virginia, he came upon a small stone church filled with badly wounded soldiers, the remnants of Union general John Pope's decimated army. The air was thick with anguished moans and the stench of putrefaction. Most of the casualties would soon die because their wounds were infected. During the Civil War, a soldier with an infected wound was doomed. "At the field hospital," one surgeon remembered, "the cases were very frequent. Statistics are unnecessary; they proved uniformly fatal." Keen believed there was a correlation between the squalid conditions in field hospitals and the staggering mortality rate of wounded soldiers, but it wasn't until Joseph Lister promulgated the germ theory of disease that Keen fully grasped the connection.

Surgery pre-Lister was a gamble that most patients were bound to lose. Even if you survived the operation itself—no mean feat, especially in the days before anesthetics—there was a better than 50 percent chance you would die of a postoperative infection. In especially unsanitary hospitals, the mortality rate often approached 100 percent. The deaths were usually attributed to "hospitalism," a vague term used to describe a variety of infections, the most prevalent and dangerous of which was gangrene. Exactly what caused hospitalism was a matter of intense and often acrimonious debate. Some doctors believed a poisonous miasma surrounded hospitals. Others believed oxygen contaminated wounds. Still others clung to the theory of spontaneous generation. The proposed cures were equally varied and fabulous. The common remedy was amputation, though this, of course, was not always feasible, and, in any event, usually led to another infection. A Scottish surgeon named James Simpson called for the abolition of hospitals altogether. He said they should be replaced with portable "villages of iron huts," which could be torn down and reassembled whenever they became infected with hospitalism.

Joseph Lister, a professor of surgery at Glasgow University, wasn't sure what to believe until 1864, when he read a paper by Louis Pasteur, who postulated that invisible organisms—germs—lived in the air and were responsible for making wine turn sour. Lister connected the dots. "It occurred to me," he wrote, "that decomposition in the injured part might be [caused by] the floating particles." By preventing germs from entering wounds, Lister believed hospitalism would be ended. Pasteur had discovered the germ theory of disease; Lister would evangelize it.

Lister began touring the world, tirelessly urging his colleagues to adopt "antiseptic" surgical practices. He told them dangerous microbes were everywhere—in the air, on their scalpels, even under their fingernails. He implored them to sanitize their operating rooms and sterilize their instruments. His pleas often fell on deaf ears. Many surgeons were loath to trade in their comfortable, crusty coats for crisp, clean smocks. Some didn't fully comprehend what Lister was getting at. If a doctor dropped a sterilized scalpel on the floor, he just picked it up and wiped it on his handkerchief. When the patient developed gangrene, he concluded that antiseptic surgery was pointless. Many doctors found Lister's claims farfetched. The editor of one medical journal huffed, "We are as likely to be as much ridiculed in the next century for our blind belief in the power of unseen germs as our forefathers were for their faith in the influence of spirits."

Lister persevered. In 1876 he traveled to Philadelphia to preach his gospel at a medical conference that was being held in conjunction with the city's Centennial Exhibition. In the audience was W. W. Keen. "I became a convert at once," Keen later wrote. After the speech Keen introduced himself to Lister. The two doctors were alike in many ways. They were both abolitionists, deeply religious but wary of fundamentalism, intensely interested in scientific research, and gifted writers. And they were both fanatical about cleanliness. They instantly became friends.

Keen immediately instituted antiseptic practices at St. Mary's Hospital, where he was then practicing. It was the first hospital in Philadelphia to follow Lister's advice. Almost overnight its postoperative mortality rate plummeted. Soon every hospital in the city followed suit. Within ten years, antiseptic surgery was practiced everywhere. Along with anesthesia, it was one of the great advances in medicine in the nineteenth century. Today the postoperative infection rate is less than 2 percent.

Joseph Lister died in 1912. Two years later his name was attached—without his family's permission—to a new brand of mouthwash. He deserves a better memorial than Listerine.

⸻ •••• ⸻

After he left the army in 1864, Keen embarked on a tour of Europe. For nearly two years he traveled the continent, from Norway to Italy, studying and sightseeing. In Vienna and Berlin, Keen studied under some of Europe's most renowned surgeons: Hyrtl, Škoda, and Virchow. In London, he watched the legendary British politicians Disraeli and Gladstone debate in the House of Commons. Though a practicing Baptist, he could not resist the urge to stand with the multitudes in St. Peter's Square on Easter Sunday 1865 and receive the blessing of Pius IX—the pope who declared popes infallible. In Paris, Keen was shown the continent's latest surgical instruments, including a cheek retractor—an ingenious device used to pull the cheek away from the jaw, allowing oral surgery to be performed wholly within the mouth. He'd never seen anything like it, so he bought one—though at the time he doubted he'd ever have much use for it.

Keen returned to Philadelphia in May 1866. He opened a private surgical practice and settled into a teaching job at Jefferson. In 1867, Tinnie Borden finally agreed to marry him, ending a courtship that had consumed eight years. Their union was productive—they had four children, all girls—but tragically abbreviated. On July 12, 1886, Tinnie suddenly died after a bout with dysentery. Keen was inconsolable; the death of his beloved wife plunged him into a crushing grief. "The one appalling disaster of my life," he called it. At thirty-nine, he was a single parent with four young daughters. His only solace was work. He spent the next year editing a new American edition of *Grey's Anatomy*, which became a standard textbook for a generation of medical students. He also edited *The American Text-book of Surgery* and *Surgery: Its Principles and Practice*, the latter being the first American textbook on surgery to incorporate Lister's antiseptic principles.

Keen also pioneered brain surgery. On December 15, 1887, he successfully removed a large tumor from the brain of a patient named Theodore Daveler—perhaps the first operation of its kind in the United States, though, in this case, the patient's resolve is at least as commendable as the surgeon's. Daveler lived another thirty years, albeit with an inch-and-a-half hole in his head protected only by a crude helmet—a skullcap fitted with a piece of tin—that Keen fashioned for him. The case cemented Keen's reputation.

Keen was pious, but he was no saint. He could be a bit overbearing—in the operating room, there were two ways to do things: his way and the wrong way. He was opinionated, too—he inundated the *Philadelphia Public Ledger* with letters to the editor. But his peers didn't seem to mind, and he had become a full-fledged member of Philadelphia's high society. He was invited to the most fashionable oyster parties. He belonged to some of the city's most prestigious and important organizations, including the American Philosophical Society and the University Club. He had succeeded Samuel Gross as the chairman of surgery at

Jefferson—and as the nation's most famous surgeon. If not the emperor of American surgery, Keen was at least a prince. His place in the pantheon was secure.

Then he got Joseph Bryant's letter.

———————————

Back on the ferry, Keen pondered Bryant's preposterous request. As Keen well knew, Grover Cleveland was not the ideal candidate for radical surgery. He was overweight and out of shape. His neck was so thick, the joke went, he could take off his shirt without unbuttoning the collar. He probably had high blood pressure. And he was exhausted. Keen knew the president might not survive the operation. The anesthesia could trigger a heart attack or stroke. It was also possible—even likely— that Cleveland would lose a large amount of blood, which, considering that no means of transfusion had yet been devised, would prove fatal.

Yet Keen did not ponder Bryant's request very long. "I readily agreed," Keen later wrote.

Although he was a rock-ribbed Republican—in 1861, as a student at Jefferson, he'd attended a speech by President-elect Abraham Lincoln at Independence Hall—Keen's respect for the presidency was nonpartisan. If the president requested his assistance, he would render it. In fact, it was Keen's policy to give aid to all who asked for it, regardless of their station. He frequently operated on indigent patients for free. Besides, Keen believed Cleveland was all that stood between "us and widespread bankruptcy."

Keen, whose passion for order and cleanliness was nearly obsessive, must have been aghast at the thought of such an important operation taking place clandestinely on a boat. But he agreed with Bryant that such secrecy was essential. "If it had been suspected that Mr. Cleveland was suffering from cancer," Keen wrote, "the possibility that his life might be shortened or his considerable influence diminished would cause the politicians to desert him (as the setting sun) and flock to the support of Stevenson (the rising sun); the Silver Act would never be repealed, and the direst possible consequences for the country would follow."

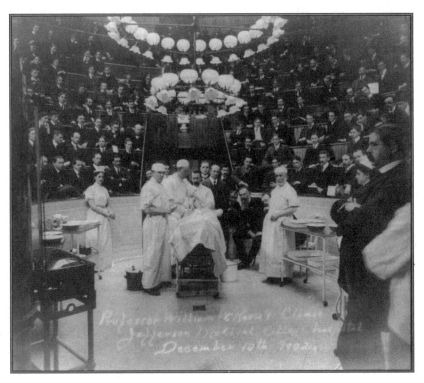

W. W. Keen in the operating theater at Jefferson Medical College, December 10, 1902. Keen is in white, standing to the right. The spectators are probably medical students. LIBRARY OF CONGRESS

By agreeing to take part in the secret operation on the president, Keen was putting his career—and his reputation—on the line. He had performed hundreds of operations but none like this. The identity of the patient and the high stakes involved would make it the most important case in American medicine since Garfield was shot twelve years earlier. And everybody knew how that turned out.

Outwardly, the president appeared remarkably calm as his appointment on the *Oneida* approached. He went about his business in his usual matter-of-fact manner. He prepared for the looming showdown with Congress over the Silver Purchase Act, vigorously lobbying representatives and senators. And he did his best to fend off the office seekers who continued to hound him.

Privately, of course, Cleveland was anxious. One senator who was friendly with the president later recalled that, at this time, "Mr. Cleveland seemed very much worried, and was continually talking about his physical condition and expressing great concern."

Robert O'Brien, who had succeeded Dan Lamont as Cleveland's private secretary, later wrote, "Mr. Cleveland had shown during the latter spring and early summer of that year a very marked tendency to get away from people, to avoid visitors, betokening some physical weariness or nervous apprehension."

In the days leading up to the operation, Dan Lamont peppered Dr. Bryant with letters and telegrams containing questions from the president. How would his speaking voice be affected? Initially he will "exhibit a defect in speech," Bryant answered. But once he was fitted with an oral prosthesis to replace the excised bits, his speaking voice should return to normal. Bryant was already in touch with Kasson Gibson, a New York dentist and prosthodontist who would go to Gray Gables after the operation to fashion an artificial jaw for the president.

The president wanted to know how soon after the operation he would be able to meet with government officials without revealing what had happened. The economic situation was dire; Cleveland was eager to set a date for the special session of Congress to convene. He preferred to summon the representatives and senators while the weather in Washington was still sultry. He hoped the heat would expedite the debate.

Bryant estimated it would take the president at least a month to recover and master the prosthesis. "When I say this I assume that everything will go as is usual in such cases," Bryant wrote. But, he warned, "Further than this, human foresight cannot indicate." If there were complications, the recovery time might be significantly longer. Bryant advised the president to schedule the special session no earlier than August 15, some six weeks after the surgery. Cleveland, of course, would be expected to return to Washington for the session. But that was not soon enough for Cleveland, Lamont wired Bryant. "Could your friend safely make engagement for seventh of August instead of fifteenth as proposed?" Reluctantly, Bryant agreed—another example of the patient, not the doctor, dictating the course of treatment.

What Bryant didn't tell the president was that, if the cancer had spread too far, the lower part of his left eye socket would have to be removed—in which case the left side of his face would droop noticeably and his vision would be permanently impaired. In that event, of course, it would be impossible to conceal the fact that the president had had major surgery.

And then there was the small matter of Cleveland's big moustache. The president undoubtedly insisted it be preserved. Even if he bore no visible scars after the operation, the sudden disappearance of his bushy 'stache would arouse intense curiosity. Indeed, at the time a clean-shaven president was almost unimaginable. There hadn't been one since Andrew Johnson left office in 1869, nearly twenty-five years earlier.

Except for some outlandish sideburns, such as those worn by John Quincy Adams and Martin Van Buren, no president sported facial hair until Abraham Lincoln, who, after his election in 1860, grew a beard at the suggestion of an eleven-year-old girl. Thereafter, excepting Johnson and McKinley, every president for the next fifty-two years was bewhiskered: Grant (beard), Hayes (beard), Garfield (beard), Arthur (moustache-meets-sideburns, a style known as the Franz Josef), Cleveland, Harrison (beard), Roosevelt (moustache), and Taft (moustache). (Although he grew a beard after his stroke, Wilson never appeared in public with it.)

How did facial hair become de rigueur for presidents? In part, the style was borrowed from British aristocrats who, by 1850, regarded shaving as "a most peculiar activity." Beards had come to be regarded as healthy. They were thought to prevent bronchitis, as well as diseases of the throat. Also, during the Civil War, most soldiers had neither the time nor the inclination to shave, and after the war they simply kept their whiskers. By 1870, facial hair had become all the rage. Even Uncle Sam, previously clean shaven, had sprouted a goatee. In a photograph of the Harvard Class of 1870, each and every graduate is sporting a beard, moustache, or some variant. Yale's yearbook that year even broke down the class by facial hair:

Moustache, 26
Sides, 19
Down (quite down), 18
Moustache and Sides, 13
Hopeful scrags, 12
Incipient hairs, 9
Moustache and Imperial, 6
Shave daily with no result, 3
Moustache and Whiskers, 3
Fuzzy in spots, 2
Feels confident that the soil is good, 1
Is applying blisters, 1

Yet, seemingly as quickly as it had become fashionable, facial hair fell out of favor. Since Taft left office in 1913, no president has had any facial hair, and only two major presidential candidates, Republicans Charles Hughes (1916) and Thomas Dewey (1944, 1948), have had any. (Hughes reportedly grew his beard to "save trips to the barber." Dewey wore a pencil-thin moustache that made him look, in the memorable words of one socialite, "like the bridegroom on the wedding cake." Although he was frequently advised to get rid of his 'stache, Dewey refused because he said his wife liked it.)

As with its ascendency, several factors contributed to facial hair's decline. In 1895, King Camp Gillette invented a disposable razor blade that made shaving easier and safer. Ironically, facial hair also came to be regarded as unhealthy. Proponents of a so-called hygiene movement postulated that beards were actually breeding grounds for "misanthropic microbes." Then came World War I. Doughboys were required to be clean shaven so their gasmasks would fit snugly. After the war came the rise of hirsute communists Lenin and Trotsky, not to mention their bearded forefathers Marx and Engels. "Facial hair had acquired a new but entirely enduring twentieth-century meaning—that of dictator, communist, or revolutionary," writes Allan Peterkin in *One Thousand Beards*, his history of facial hair. "The beard has been the kiss of death for Western politicians ever since."

Though he regarded communism as "a hateful thing and a menace to peace," Grover Cleveland was fond of his furry upper lip and was loath to lose it. He'd first grown his moustache as a young man back in Buffalo and can be seen sporting it in the first known photograph of him, taken in 1864, when he was twenty-seven. His moustache had become his trademark.

―――――――

On June 26, the same day he met Dr. Keen on the ferry, Joseph Bryant also convinced another prominent doctor to join the secret surgical team. Like Bryant, fifty-two-year-old Edward Janeway was a former New York City health commissioner and a professor at Bellevue Hospital Medical College. Also like Bryant, he was an accomplished surgeon.

That night, Bryant returned to his handsome home at 54 West Thirty-Sixth Street and wrote a letter to Dan Lamont in Washington. "My dear Col.," the letter begins,

> My arrangements are now all but complete. I saw the gentleman from Philadelphia today. He will accompany us.
>
> Now Col., if you do not intend that Dr. O'R. [O'Reilly, the White House physician] go along, for politic or other reasons, then you should let me know at once, for I must then find someone else. It is my intention to give the anesthetic myself until time to begin the operation. I do this because I can thus set the example, and also perhaps the patient will regard it with some degree of satisfaction. However, someone must begin when I leave off, and I had assigned Dr. O'R. to this duty, as I cannot expect either of the other gentlemen [Keen and Janeway] to do this for many good reasons. Telegraph me when you leave.
>
> Do you not think that there should be a "cipher" code, which can be used? It seems to me that this will be especially important in case anything unfavorable happens. If anything "springs a leak"

it may not be amiss. Tell our friend [the president] that I desire his
urine examined two or three times before leaving for here. B. [Elias
Benedict, owner of the *Oneida*] is entering into this matter with
earnest and well-directed zeal. Does the wife know about it? I ask
because she may write me and I wish to know what to say. Give my
regards to the President.

A cipher was never used; although, considering Bryant's abstruse
wording and abysmal penmanship, it hardly seems to have been
warranted.

In the end, it was decided that O'Reilly should be included on
the surgical team, and in the following days, two more doctors were
recruited: John Erdmann, Bryant's twenty-nine-year-old assistant and
protégé, and Ferdinand Hasbrouck, a forty-nine-year-old dentist who
was also an experienced anesthetist. Born in Monticello, New York,
around 1843, Hasbrouck was one of the first dentists to experiment
with anesthesia, and he built a thriving practice in New York City, earning a reputation that "brought many noted people as patients." In 1892
the *New York Press* called Hasbrouck "the most expert tooth extractor in
the world" and estimated that he had pulled seventy thousand teeth.
Since Cleveland's tumor was very close to his molars, some of his teeth
would need to be extracted. When Joseph Bryant was assembling his
surgical team, Hasbrouck, with his expertise in dentistry as well as anesthesia, was a logical choice. However, Hasbrouck's services were very
much in demand, and he already had an appointment to assist a doctor named Carlos MacDonald with an operation in Greenwich the day
after the operation on the *Oneida*. Hasbrouck told Bryant he would need
to disembark soon after the surgery on the president had ended.

The surgical team was now complete: Bryant would be the lead
surgeon; Keen and Erdmann would assist. Hasbrouck would handle
tooth extractions and assist with anesthesia. O'Reilly would also assist
with anesthesia, and Janeway would monitor the patient's vital signs. All
were sworn to secrecy.

Meanwhile, Bryant oversaw preparations on the *Oneida*, which Benedict had anchored in the East River that week. The yacht's small, dark saloon was transformed into a makeshift operating room. It was cleared of all furniture except the organ, which was bolted to the floor. Then it was cleaned and disinfected. A large chair was lashed to the mast in the center of the room. Here the president would sit for the operation. There would be no operating table. The only artificial light would come from a single electric bulb connected to a portable battery. The larger pieces of equipment, including tanks of oxygen and nitrous oxide, were quietly delivered to the yacht. Regarding the unusual accumulation of medical paraphernalia, Dr. Keen later said the crew of the *Oneida* was told "that the president had to have two very badly ulcerated teeth removed and that fresh, pure air, and disinfected quarters and skilled doctors, all had to be provided, lest blood poisoning should set in—a very serious matter when the patient was the just-inaugurated President of the United States." It would later be reported that the white yacht was repainted green in order to better conceal it, but that was not true. As Elias Benedict himself later noted, "Such an act would have created a suspicion which we all wished to avoid." The intent, of course, was to make it look like a perfectly ordinary summer outing for the president and his friends.

5

THE *ONEIDA*

O N FRIDAY, JUNE 30, 1893, President Cleveland awoke around
seven and read the morning papers over his usual breakfast of
beefsteak and eggs. The headlines must have troubled him as greatly
as the rough spot on the roof of his mouth. They told of more failed
banks, more closed mines, more foreclosed farms, and more bankrupt
businesses. Wheat prices were at an all-time low: seventy cents a bushel.
Interest rates on Wall Street were at an all-time high: 74 percent. Stocks
were plummeting accordingly.

But amid the tales of financial disaster in the papers that morning
were stories reflecting the almost naïve optimism of what has come to be
called the Gilded Age.* Arctic explorer Robert Peary was on his way to
Greenland for the second time. The massive engines of the navy's new-
est battleship, the *Maine*, were successfully tested at the Brooklyn Navy
Yard. At the World's Fair in Chicago, final preparations were underway

---

* The moniker Gilded Age was popularized by Mark Twain, who intended it as an epithet: to gild
was to be obnoxiously extravagant.

for the grandest Fourth of July celebration ever. And excited crowds were packing National League ballparks, eager to see the results of the new, longer distance between the pitcher's mound and home plate: sixty feet, six inches. They rarely went home disappointed. Batting averages rose faster than interest rates.*

As far as Grover Cleveland was concerned, though, the best news in the papers that day came from an unlikely source: his old foe, Benjamin Harrison. Speaking to reporters in New York, the former president announced his support for repealing the Sherman Silver Purchase Act, which he had signed into law three years before. Harrison conceded that repealing the act would have a positive effect on public opinion, which he held responsible for the crumbling economy: "I do not attribute all of the evils of the present financial situation to the Sherman Act, but in the imagination of the people; that is one strong cause, and so I believe that its repeal would be beneficial." It was feeble affirmation, but it was good enough for Cleveland, who had won a symbolically important, if grudging, ally. For the first time in weeks, he must have put the morning papers down with a smile.

That morning, Cleveland worked feverishly to clear his desk—literally. The president did not share W. W. Keen's "love of order." His massive *Resolute* desk was always covered with piles of paper. As president, he was required to personally sign a mountain of documents every day—military commissions, land grants, diplomatic correspondence. Cleveland never learned how to properly dictate to a stenographer, so he answered in his own hand every letter he received, no matter how mundane. He also wrote drafts of his speeches in longhand. The piles on his desk occasionally grew tall enough to obscure the enormous president behind them. Now facing an extended "vacation," Cleveland was eager to leave behind as little work as possible.

Later that day, Cleveland signed the commissions of four naval cadets, including the first two to be trained in steam engineering.

---

* Grover was a baseball fan but never attended a game as president. "What do you imagine the American people would think of me if I wasted my time going to the ball game?" he rhetorically asked the Chicago White Stockings star Cap Anson in 1885.

He also signed the proclamation summoning Congress for a special session to consider repealing the Silver Purchase Act. The lawmakers were to convene on August 7. It would be just the eleventh special session ever called by a president. In a draft of the proclamation, War Secretary Dan Lamont scribbled in the margin: "Written the day the president left Washington on account of illness." Lamont, of course, was the only member of Cleveland's cabinet aware of the impending operation.

Around four o'clock that afternoon, Cleveland and Lamont climbed into the White House carriage and rode down Pennsylvania Avenue to the Baltimore and Potomac train station, where Garfield had been shot twelve years earlier.* No bodyguards accompanied them. The Secret Service would not begin protecting presidents until the following year, when agents uncovered a plot by a group of gamblers in Colorado to assassinate Cleveland, perhaps at the behest of pro-silver forces.

At the station they boarded a special Pullman that was attached to the end of the Pennsylvania Railroad's New York Express. The Pullman belonged to Frank Thompson, the railroad's vice president, who, at Lamont's request, had loaned it to the president "with the greatest pleasure." Inside the car, Cleveland ordered the curtains drawn. He took off his heavy Prince Albert jacket and unbuttoned his collar. His heavily starched shirt was soaked with sweat. Exhausted, he threw himself into an upholstered chair and demanded a whiskey and a cigar, which a dutiful porter promptly produced.

The train pulled out at 4:20 P.M.—right on time. The president's departure was unannounced. By the time reporters in the capital learned that he'd called a special session of Congress, he was already gone.

Lamont did not disturb the president, who stared out the window, silently watching Washington melt into Maryland through a cloud of tobacco smoke. Every few miles the train passed a shantytown along the tracks, each populated by the victims of the Panic of 1893. They were known as the mudsill—the lowest of the low. Too poor even to afford the meager rents of tenements, they roamed the cities and countryside

---

* The station was demolished in 1908. The National Archives is now on the site.

by the thousands: homeless, jobless, hungry, and desperate. "Men died like flies under the strain," wrote nineteenth- and early-twentieth-century historian Henry Adams of the panic. Some families were reduced to eating grass.

The president didn't have to worry about eating grass, but he certainly had his own concerns, even beyond his grave executive responsibilities. Office seekers still hounded him. His wife's pregnancy—Frances was now due to give birth in two months—preoccupied him. And he had cancer. In less than twenty-four hours he would undergo radical surgery to remove the tumor in his mouth.

He still sat in silence, gazing out the window of the speeding Pullman, hurtling toward New York at a mile a minute. His only consolation was that not a word of his condition had leaked. The papers were oblivious to his impending operation. For that, at least, he was grateful.

Maryland gave way to Delaware. Wilmington approached. He demanded another whiskey.

Meanwhile, the five doctors who would assist Bryant in the operation the next day quietly gathered on the *Oneida*. Erdmann, Hasbrouck, Janeway, Keen, and O'Reilly were each ferried to the yacht from different piers in the *Oneida*'s naphtha launch, an early version of a motorboat with a notoriously unpredictable engine. O'Reilly had traveled to New York incognito under the pseudonym Major Miller.

At 10:32 P.M., the president's train pulled into Jersey City. Dr. Bryant was waiting for him. So were several reporters, but Cleveland was in no mood for them. On the ferry from Jersey City to Manhattan—the panic had put an end to dreams of building a tunnel under the Hudson—he growled at a *New York Times* correspondent, "I have nothing to say for publication, except that I am going to Buzzards Bay for a rest." It was the first of many half-truths, exaggerations, and outright lies that the press would be told about the operation.

The ferry ride took about twenty minutes, after which Cleveland, Lamont, and Bryant squeezed into Bryant's landau and rode, unnoticed in the darkness, across Lower Manhattan to Pier A on the East River. The *Oneida* was anchored a good distance offshore to keep prying eyes

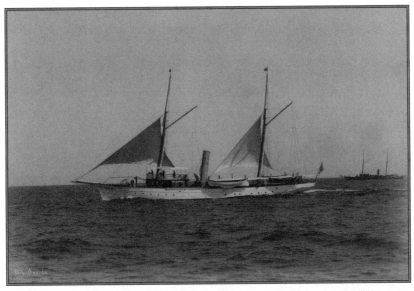

The *Oneida* was one of the most spectacular yachts of the Gilded Age. Though not exceptionally large, the boat was fast and luxurious. HISTORIC NEW ENGLAND

at bay. The naphtha launch was waiting to shuttle the three men to the yacht.

Even by the Gilded Age's gaudy standards, the *Oneida* was a fabulous boat. Built in 1883 and originally christened the *Utowana*, the yacht won the Lunberg Cup, an international race, in 1885. So impressed was Elias Benedict, a fanatical yachtsman, that he bought the boat, refitted it for comfort as well as speed, and renamed it the *Oneida*, perhaps to honor the first tribe to side with the Americans in the Revolutionary War. At 138 feet the *Oneida* wasn't exceptionally large (J. P. Morgan's yacht was more than twice as long), but it was fast and luxurious, capable of running thirteen knots and comfortably accommodating a dozen passengers. It had an iron hull, two masts, and a steam engine. The quarters below deck were plush, though, by necessity, somewhat cramped. The *Oneida* combined the elegance of a schooner, the speed of a steamer, and the comfort of a luxury liner. It had been built in Chester, Pennsylvania, by John Roach, a brilliant, self-educated Irish immigrant who pioneered iron shipbuilding in the United States. Besides building yachts for the rich and famous, including almost-president Samuel Tilden, he also built the U.S. Navy's first fleet of modern warships. Roach died in 1887—of cancer of the mouth.

On the deck of the yacht, the president met with the doctors who would operate on him the next day. He already knew Bryant and O'Reilly, of course, and he'd almost certainly met Erdmann, Bryant's assistant, as well. But Cleveland had probably never before been introduced to the other three doctors, Hasbrouck, Janeway, and Keen.

Grover sat in a deck chair, lit a cigar, and chatted with the doctors for about thirty minutes. For the first time all day he seemed relaxed. It was one of those increasingly rare moments when the other Grover emerged, the jovial raconteur. The warm night air was filled with pleasant chatter and the sweet smell of fine cigars. At one point Grover burst out, "Those officeseekers! They haunt me even in my dreams!" Around midnight the group retired to their cabins, except Bryant and Lamont, who returned to their respective homes in Manhattan. (Lamont maintained homes in both Washington and New York.) Dr. Keen later reported that the president needed no sedatives and slept soundly through the night, office-seeker dreams notwithstanding.

One wonders how soundly the doctors slept.

Cleveland was awakened the next morning by a knock on his cabin door. Begging his pardon, Janeway asked the president if he could examine him before he dressed. Grover consented unenthusiastically. His ambivalence toward doctors was well known. To an ailing friend he once wrote, "I hope that either by following your doctor's directions or defiantly disobeying them (the chances probably being even in both contingencies), you will soon regain your very best estate in the matter of health."

Janeway found the president to be in surprisingly good shape. He was overweight, but his heart and lungs were healthy. He had little if any hardening of the arteries and no enlarged glands. His pulse was ninety beats per minute.

Janeway washed out the president's mouth with a disinfectant called Thiersch's solution and declared him fit for the operation.

Keen also examined the president that morning, personally inspecting the tumor for the first time. It was even larger than he'd expected. The grayish growth covered much of the left side of the palate. The surface was rough and cauliflowerlike. It looked like a giant wart.

When he concluded his examination of the president, Keen was troubled by just one thing: a urinalysis revealed early-stage chronic nephritis, a kidney disease that is often dangerously aggravated by ether. The question of anesthesia vexed the doctors greatly. Keen held out hope that the entire operation could be performed with nitrous oxide, thereby avoiding ether altogether. Nitrous oxide (N_2O), or laughing gas, was a popular recreational drug until its anesthetic properties were discovered by a Hartford dentist named Horace Wells in 1844. It was considerably less powerful than ether, which made it difficult to use in long operations, but it was also much safer, since ether frequently triggered pneumonia and other side effects. Ether was also highly combustible, an especially grave concern in a confined, poorly ventilated space—such as the saloon

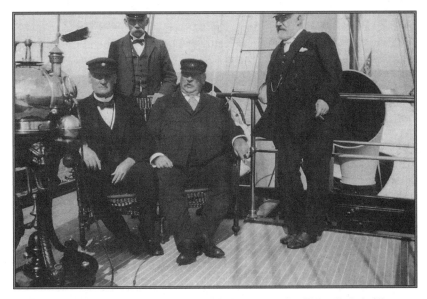

Grover Cleveland (seated right) and "Commodore" Elias Benedict (standing right) on the deck of the *Oneida* in 1898, five years after the operation. NEW JERSEY STATE PARK SERVICE; PHOTO RESTORATION BY AL J. FRAZZA

of a yacht. Like Keen, Bryant had hoped to "do this job with the use of laughing gas." But Hasbrouck, the dentist who was also an experienced anesthetist, didn't think nitrous oxide would be strong enough for the Cleveland surgery. "In the use of nitrous oxide for the operation about to be made," he wrote in his case notes, "it is very doubtful in my opinion about keeping him under the influence of it for a sufficient length of time to complete the various steps of the operation as explained to me." The doctors compromised: they would begin the operation with nitrous oxide and switch to ether only if absolutely necessary.

The preoperative examinations complete, Grover dressed in his usual dark suit and joined Commodore Benedict on the deck for a leisurely breakfast. They were joined by Bryant and Lamont, who had returned from their homes. The mood was relaxed, but the president's famously voracious appetite was absent. He had only coffee and toast, though even that was too much. Surgical patients today are instructed to fast immediately before an operation, to minimize the risk of vomiting and possibly choking while anesthetized.

After breakfast, it was solemnly noted, the president "moved his bladder and bowels in a natural manner."

Benedict ordered anchors aweigh, and the *Oneida* began steaming up the East River at half speed. It was a clear, bright Saturday morning, and the water was crowded with ferries and trawlers and schooners and even a few other yachts, but they all made way for the majestic *Oneida*, its spotless white hull gleaming in the fetid water. Like a bride gliding down the aisle, the boat effortlessly sailed the narrow channel between Manhattan and Queens. Cleveland, Benedict, Bryant, and Lamont sat casually on the deck chatting, looking to all the world like four carefree gentlemen on a pleasure cruise. On both shores, crowds gathered to catch a glimpse of the grand yacht and its esteemed passengers.

The rest of the surgical team was hidden from view. "Passing the foot of 56th Street opposite Bellevue Hospital," Dr. Erdmann remembered, "Dr. Bryant was particularly careful that we on board should not be recognized by any of the staff of Bellevue Hospital looking out. We went into the cabin so that we should not be recognized."

After navigating the treacherous currents of the Hell Gate, the *Oneida* turned eastward and headed for the cleaner, bluer, bigger waters of Long Island Sound. The weather was perfect, and, much to everyone's relief, the water was calm. As the *Oneida* entered the sound, the mood on board turned more serious. When Bryant excused himself to join the other doctors below deck, he called out to the captain jokingly, "If you hit a rock, hit it good and hard, so that we'll all go to the bottom!" Nobody laughed.

In the saloon, the six doctors made final preparations for the operation. Quietly they washed their hands. Adhering strictly to Lister's advice, they sterilized their instruments by boiling them in water. They pulled crisp white aprons over their dark suits.

The doctors would be assisted by Charles Peterson, the *Oneida*'s "extremely loyal and faithful" chief steward, who would fetch hot water, towels, and bandages as needed.

It's worth mentioning just a few of the tools that the surgeons would not have at their disposal, simply because they had not yet been devised or perfected. They would have no suction apparatus for draining blood and other fluids from the operative site and no means of artificially resuscitating the patient should his heart stop. There would be no electronic monitors, no ventilators, no laryngoscopes, no endotracheal tubes. Surgery had come a long way since the Civil War—but it still had a long way to go.

Shortly after noon, Cleveland returned to his cabin and stripped to his underwear. Then he walked into the saloon cum operating room. All but naked, the president of the United States stood before the surgeons in whose hands he now placed his life. He was calm, Keen remembered. It was a scene unprecedented in American history. Yes, presidents had undergone surgery before. Just six weeks into his first term, Washington had had a large carbuncle—a benign tumor—removed from his thigh without the benefit of painkillers. But never before had a president submitted willingly to a radical operation under anesthesia.

Cleveland took his seat in the operating chair. His legs were stretched out, and his head was tilted back, as if he were trying to catch a nap.

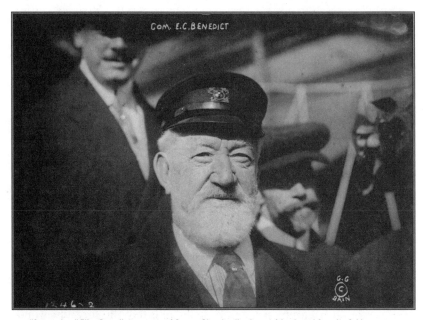

"Commodore" Elias Benedict was one of Grover Cleveland's closest friends and favorite fishing partners. It was on his yacht that the president's secret operation took place. LIBRARY OF CONGRESS

Pillows tied to the chair helped hold him in position. The doctors and Charles Peterson, the steward, took their places around the patient. No one else was in the room. Lamont and Benedict stayed up on the deck, lounging conspicuously, struggling to project an air of nonchalance to passing boats.

Keen, ever the devout Baptist, offered a brief prayer, and at thirty-two minutes after noon Hasbrouck put a mask to the president's face and began administering nitrous oxide. As Cleveland inhaled the gas, his hands trembled and twitched, but he didn't succumb. Hasbrouck had to give him a second dose, and it took four minutes for the president to be sufficiently anesthetized. Keen's heart sank. Hasbrouck had been right. Clearly, nitrous oxide would not be strong enough for the whole operation. At some point, ether would have to be administered.

It had been decided that the president's two left upper bicuspids should be removed first. With a pair of dental pliers, Hasbrouck expertly extracted each tooth with a sharp yank. The president began to bleed. The hemorrhaging was stopped with manual pressure and an electric cautery, a device that sealed the wound by burning it. The scent of seared flesh began to fill the saloon. "Pulse remained first rate," O'Reilly noted. "No pain."

A cocaine solution was injected around the edges of the tumor; at 12:50 P.M., more gas was administered.

Using what was essentially a small electric carving knife, Bryant began making an incision around the tumor, cutting through the soft palate and the gums. Suddenly, Janeway noticed that the president seemed to be regaining consciousness. Frantically, Hasbrouck grabbed the mask and pressed it to Cleveland's face, swiftly administering yet another dose of nitrous oxide. Assured the president was anesthetized once more, Bryant quickly finished the incision.

It was now time for what Keen called "the more severe and bloody part" of the operation: the removal of the affected bone and tissue. For this there was now no question that ether would have to be administered. Keen murmured another short prayer as O'Reilly carefully placed the mask of the ether inhaler over the president's mouth and nose.

At 1:14 P.M., Bryant began to remove the tumor. Using the ingenious little retractor that Keen had bought in Paris nearly thirty years earlier, Bryant pulled back the president's left cheek and, using a small scalpel, he cut the fleshy jowl away from the upper jaw. Then he began removing part of the president's upper left jaw. "The front of the jaw was then chiseled loose from the first bicuspid to the posterior extremity of the bone," Keen noted. Then, with a pair of heavy forceps, known as a ronguer, Bryant removed the affected parts of the president's hard palate. Three more teeth were also removed. All the excised matter was carefully placed in a small jar.

At this point the surgeons discovered just how far the cancer seemed to have spread. The antrum—the cavity above the roof of the mouth—was filled with what Keen described as a "gelatinous mass . . . totally different in appearance from the typical epithelioma of the roof of the mouth." Bryant gingerly scooped out the gelatinous substance with a small spoon.

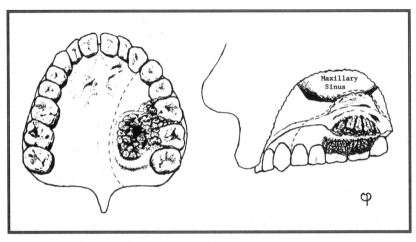

This drawing, originally published in *Transactions & Studies of the College of Physicians of Philadelphia*, depicts the tumor as it appeared in the president's mouth. The dotted line corresponds to the area that was removed during the operation. COURTESY OF THE HISTORICAL MEDICAL LIBRARY OF THE COLLEGE OF PHYSICIANS OF PHILADELPHIA

Fortunately for the president, his eye socket was "clearly free from invasion."

The doctors disinfected the wound with Thiersch's solution and packed it with gauze.

At 1:55 P.M. the operation was over. It had taken nearly an hour and a half. Five teeth, about a third of the upper palate, and a large piece of the upper left jawbone had been removed. The resulting cavity was two and a half inches long and nearly an inch wide. The president's pulse

This laryngeal mirror and cheek retractor were used in the secret surgery on President Cleveland. Dr. William Williams Keen had bought the unusual retractor in Paris nearly thirty years before the operation. MÜTTER MUSEUM OF THE COLLEGE OF PHYSICIANS OF PHILADELPHIA

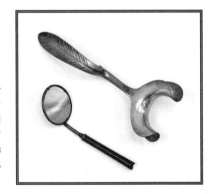

had fallen to eighty. His temperature was 100.8 degrees. He'd lost at least six ounces of blood—and, of course, had received none in transfusion. But he was still alive.

"Never did I feel such a deep, almost overwhelming, sense of responsibility as during that operation," Keen wrote years later. "In itself, it was nothing as compared with many others I have done of greater difficulty and danger, but in its possible consequences for good or evil, none I ever was involved in could compare with it."

The nation, of course, was utterly ignorant of the drama that unfolded on the *Oneida* that afternoon. If they thought about him at all, Americans assumed their president was just going up to Buzzards Bay for a little rest and relaxation. That's what he'd told them.

In fact, at the very moment President Cleveland was slumped, unconscious, in a makeshift operating room on board a moving boat on Long Island Sound, the nation's attention was fixed on the opposite end of New York State. A steeplejack and tightrope walker from Ontario named Clifford Calverly was attempting to cross a wire strung over Niagara Falls. Ten months earlier Calverly had made the trip on a three-quarter-inch steel cable in a record-shattering two minutes and thirty-two seconds. This time his pace was more leisurely. At one point the daring funambulist skipped rope on the taut wire two hundred feet above the roiling water. Then he brought a chair out, sat down, and—as if all that weren't dangerous enough—he smoked a cigarette. His feats rivaled those of Jean Francois Gravelot, a.k.a. the Great Blondin, a Frenchman who crossed the gorge on a tightrope more than a dozen times in 1859 and 1860, once with his manager on his back. Calverly's manager wasn't on his back—at least not literally—but his act, according to one report, "caused the immense throng of people who lined the bridges and banks of the river to catch their breath with astonishment and fear."

Yet even Clifford Calverly's extraordinary exploits paled in comparison to the secret proceedings on the *Oneida*.

At 2:25 P.M., the president began to regain consciousness. Understandably, he complained of pain. He was given a shot of morphine. Then the doctors half carried, half dragged the enormous, groggy, almost-naked chief executive to his cabin. Keen recalled, "What a sigh of intense relief we surgeons breathed when the patient was once more safe in bed can hardly be imagined!" Of course, Cleveland wasn't out of the woods yet. It remained to be seen whether the ether would aggravate his kidney condition or trigger side effects. And other postoperative complications—blood poisoning, localized infection—were quite possible. The doctors still weren't certain he would survive.

Nonetheless, by any measure, the operation had been a success. Not only had Cleveland pulled through, but the surgery had taken place entirely within his mouth, without any external incisions. The president's eyeball hadn't been displaced. His moustache was intact. When the swelling subsided and he was fitted with an oral prosthesis, his appearance would be perfectly normal. And once he mastered the prosthesis that would be inserted in his mouth—and if everybody else kept their mouths shut—the deception would be complete. No one would ever know what really happened on the *Oneida*.

Cleveland spent the rest of the day in his cabin, drifting in and out of consciousness. The doctors took turns at his bedside, watching his vital signs and reading to him to pass the time. At one point the disoriented president looked up to see Dr. Erdmann at his bedside and demanded to know what was going on. Satisfied with the explanation that he was recovering from surgery, Cleveland then asked Erdmann where he was from.

"Chillicothe," the doctor replied.

"Oh," said the president with great difficulty. "Do you know a Mr. Nigbe there?"

"Yes, he's the druggist."

"Well, is he so poor that he needs a job from me?"

"No."

"Then he won't get one!"

With the gauze packed into the wound in his mouth, Cleveland's speech was barely intelligible. When the packing was removed, it was utterly incomprehensible, resembling, in Keen's words, "the worst imaginable case of cleft palate."

Late that afternoon, Dr. Hasbrouck asked to be let off the yacht at New London, Connecticut. He had an important appointment in Greenwich the next day, and if he wasn't put ashore by nightfall, he'd never make it on time. His request was denied. Bryant deemed it far too risky. Cleveland's condition was still precarious. Hasbrouck's services would be needed if another operation was necessary overnight. And if the yacht ran aground or hit a rock while docking, the jolt might trigger a hemorrhage or a stroke. Besides, Bryant feared suspicions would be aroused if the *Oneida* docked unexpectedly.

Hasbrouck was irate. When he'd agreed to assist in the president's surgery, he'd told Bryant about the operation in Greenwich. But Bryant was adamant. Hasbrouck would not be put ashore at New London until the next morning.

By the evening Cleveland's condition was stable. His pulse improved to ninety, and his fever subsided. The doctors, tired and hungry, took a light supper on the deck while the steward watched over the president. Afterward, cigars were passed out, and a bottle of whiskey was uncorked. (Keen abstained from the latter.) The weather, which had so far cooperated magnificently, was turning. A cool breeze blew, and high clouds raced across the nearly full moon. The flickering lights of New London were barely visible on the horizon. The *Oneida* moved in big lazy circles on the sound, in a holding pattern until Hasbrouck was let off in the morning. Bryant pulled out the small glass jar containing the matter removed from the president and held it up for all to see. The doctors began discussing its pathology. They agreed that it appeared to be an epithelioma, the same form of cancer that had killed General Grant. But the gelatinous mass from the president's antrum puzzled them; it seemed to be a different type of cancer altogether.

One of the doctors also pointed out a curious characteristic of the tumor: it had perforated the president's palate. In other words, it had grown *through* it, not simply on it. An uncomfortable silence befell the deck. Everyone knew what that meant: a tumor that perforates tissue can be a symptom of syphilis.

The conversation quickly turned lighter.

Around ten o'clock the doctors went to bed and, presumably, slept quite well.

———————————

Early the next morning, July 2, Hasbrouck was landed at New London without incident. That afternoon the president was feeling much better. He even managed to get out of bed and walk a bit. By the next day, July 3, he was "up and about," according to Keen. He was even strong enough to climb the narrow staircase to the deck, where he signed the ship's register.

On July 4, 1893, Americans did their best to celebrate Independence Day, despite the country's financial troubles. At the World's Fair, a crowd of one hundred thousand was enthralled by the most magnificent display of fireworks in memory, launched from boats anchored in Lake Michigan. Philadelphia—which had lent the Liberty Bell to Chicago for the fair—held "patriotic exercises" at Independence Hall and a regatta on the Schuylkill. In New York, police bemoaned the growing popularity of firecrackers. "Crackers are getting more dangerous for children to play with every year," a Sergeant Walsh lamented. At Niagara Falls, Clifford Calverly marked the occasion by crossing the gorge after dark, setting off Roman candles along the way.

All that was missing was Grover Cleveland.

Incredibly, the president's whereabouts were unknown on the Fourth of July. He hadn't been seen or heard from in three days. Usually, it only took the *Oneida* fifteen hours or so to get from New York to Buzzards Bay. Naturally, the reporters assigned to cover Cleveland's arrival at Gray Gables began to get curious. About eight reporters had been sent to the president's summer home, mostly from the larger daily papers in Boston and New York. They were staying at Walker's, a hotel near the Buzzards Bay railroad depot, about a mile and a half down the road from Gray Gables and not far from the town of Bourne. Privately, some began to speculate that the president was unwell. After all, he had been looking awfully haggard lately. Publicly, though, there was nothing to report but the banal speculations of locals. Under the headline "No

Sign of the *Oneida*," the *New York Times* correspondent reported that "it is the opinion here that the yacht is at anchor down the bay awaiting the clearing of the thick fog, which will allow her to proceed." The changing weather had given Cleveland the perfect cover.

On the whole, the papers regarded the president's disappearance with remarkable insouciance. The *Times*' bland report was buried on page five and was considerably shorter than an adjacent story about the arrival of Jefferson Davis's widow, Varina Howell Davis, in Rhode Island for her summer holiday. The scant attention paid the chief executive's extended absence illustrates just how superfluous the presidency was in 1893. A succession of relatively weak, ineffective presidents—Hayes, Garfield, Arthur, and Harrison—had practically emasculated the office. Cleveland had done his best to wrest control of the government from an all-powerful Congress—he was the first president to invoke executive privilege, and, as we have seen, he was unafraid to exercise his power to veto bills he found objectionable. But he never really succeeded in restoring vigor to the presidency, which may explain why his disappearance seems to have sparked more curiosity than concern.

Still, even in 1893, it was rather unusual for the president to go missing.

Late on the night of July 4, the *Oneida* anchored about two miles off Sag Harbor, on the eastern end of Long Island. In the darkness, Erdmann, Janeway, Keen, and O'Reilly were put ashore in the naphtha launch. Bryant rode along to fetch some supplies for the yacht.

And then the *Oneida* slipped back into the darkness and fog.

PART II

THE SCOOP

6

THE COVER-UP

B UILT ON MONUMENT POINT, a small peninsula jutting into Buzzards Bay on the western end of Cape Cod, Gray Gables was frequently called a cottage, but it was actually an imposing, three-story, gray-shingled mansion with eight gables and a wraparound porch. A massive stone fireplace dominated the main parlor, where the Clevelands frequently entertained. Grover had first come to the area in the summer of 1889. The journalist Richard Gilder, one of Grover's friends from New York, kept a summer home on the bay, and he invited the then-former president up to do a little fishing. It was love at first cast. Grover found the fishing so exceptional—the bay was thick with bluefish and sea bass—that he returned the following summer and, in 1891, bought Gray Gables.

Besides Gilder, several other friends from New York kept summer homes nearby, including actor Joseph Jefferson, journalist L. Clarke Davis, and Commodore Elias Benedict. In fact, it was at a party at Gilder's home that Grover first met Benedict, who remembered the occasion this way: "Toward the middle of the evening two strangers entered, one rather short, but the other a very powerfully built figure, and dressed in a manner somewhat in contrast to the rather summery garments of the others present. . . . A moment later I was shaking hands with Grover Cleveland. The shorter man was Dan Lamont." Cleveland and Benedict discovered they had much in common: both had come of age in Buffalo, both were fanatical fishermen, and both were sons of Presbyterian ministers. "We . . . found to our delight," Benedict said, "that we had both suffered in about the same measure from the severity of the Calvinistic Puritanical atmosphere which had surrounded our boyish days." They soon became a fixture on the bay, their lines trailing behind the *Oneida*, with Grover in a floppy straw hat and the commodore in a captain's cap.

Some of the best times of Grover's life were spent at Gray Gables. In the company of his friends around the big fireplace or out on the porch, the raconteur of old would return. With a cigar in one hand and a whiskey in the other, he was the life of the party. "With a few familiar friends," Richard Gilder wrote, "he was the soul of good company; not dominating the conversation, but doing his share of repartee and storytelling, with all the aids of wit, a good memory for detail, and, when necessary, the faculty of mimicry." Joseph Jefferson liked to tell Grover he'd gone into the wrong profession; he should have been an actor.

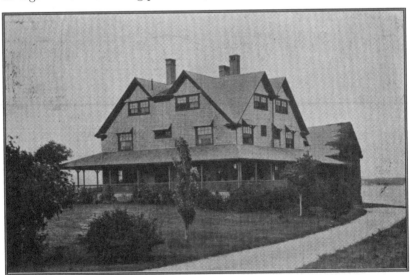

Gray Gables was the Cleveland family's summer home on Buzzards Bay in Massachusetts. Often referred to as a cottage, it was actually a three-story mansion. It was here that Grover came to recuperate after his secret operation on the *Oneida*. AUTHOR'S COLLECTION

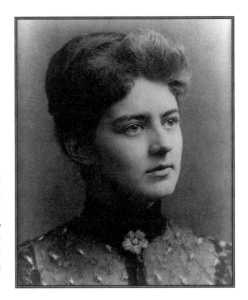

Frances Folsom Cleveland, photographed around 1886, the year she married Grover. At twenty-one, Frances was the youngest First Lady in American history. In the summer of 1893 she also became the first incumbent First Lady known to be pregnant. LIBRARY OF CONGRESS

But there would be no witty repartee on this visit to Gray Gables. Grover would barely be able to speak.

While the *Oneida* bobbed aimlessly in the foggy waters of the bay, Frances Cleveland waited anxiously inside the big gray house. It had been two weeks since she'd met with Dr. Bryant in New York to discuss the peculiar lesion in her husband's mouth. Then she'd come up to Gray Gables to wait for Grover to join her. Frances knew an operation was taking place on the *Oneida*, and though Grover tried to downplay the seriousness of it, she was rightly concerned. Wireless telegraphy was still a gleam in Marconi's eye, so there was no way for Frances to receive any information directly from the yacht. Perhaps Keen or one of the other doctors sent her a message after disembarking, but even then she would have received only the sketchiest of details. Not until she saw Grover with her own eyes would she know his true condition. It must have been an excruciating vigil. Yet, for the secret to be kept, it was imperative for her to project an air of casual indifference. On the morning of July 4, some papers reported that Mrs. Cleveland was worried about the president's absence. Some even suggested the president was seriously ill. Among doctors in New York, there was even a rumor circulating that the president had had a tumor removed from his mouth. Inevitably this rumor made its way into the pages of the more sensational papers.

That afternoon, Frances telephoned the reporters waiting at Walker's hotel and asked them to refrain from publishing any more "disquieting stories" about the president. She explained that there was no mystery about his whereabouts: he was fishing, and he "intended to take his time and stay as long on the way as the fishing would warrant." Local anglers said the bluefish were expected to return to the bay any day. The president, Frances insisted, "was well and in good health."

Frances was now seven months pregnant, and her condition was plainly visible. The newspapers noted the fact, of course, but always obliquely. Like "cancer," "pregnant" was not a word suited for proper newspapers. Instead, readers were told of Mrs. Cleveland's "expected illness." Never before had an incumbent First Lady been known to be pregnant, and the birth of the Clevelands' second child was anticipated even more eagerly than the birth of Baby Ruth. Frances's pregnancy was a rare burst of sunshine in what was turning out to be a stormy year.

With a toddler and an ailing husband to look after, the expectant Frances would have her hands full at Gray Gables. For help she summoned the president's sister, Mary Hoyt, who lived in Beatrice, Nebraska. Mrs. Hoyt's sudden departure for Gray Gables fueled more speculation about the president's health.

The *Oneida* finally reached Gray Gables on the night of Wednesday, July 5—more than four days after leaving New York. Cleveland, accompanied by Bryant and Lamont, took the launch to a small dock on the property. According to Bryant—hardly an impartial observer—the president was able to "walk sharply from the launch to his residence with but little apparent effort." The *Oneida*, with Benedict on board, anchored off Monument Point for the night and, early the next morning, set sail for the trip back to New York.

Conveniently, the president had arrived at such a late hour that the handful of reporters assigned to Gray Gables were back at the hotel and not present to witness his landing. The next morning, when they learned of the president's late-night arrival, the reporters were irate. To

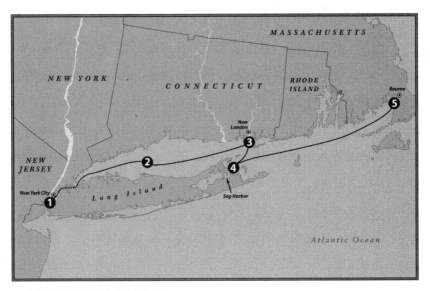

ROUTE OF THE ONEIDA, JULY 1–5, 1893

1. July 1, A.M. Departs New York City
2. July 1, P.M. Operation performed, Long Island Sound
3. July 2, A.M. Dr. Hasbrouck disembarks, New London, Connecticut
4. July 4, P.M. Anchors off Sag Harbor, Long Island; Drs. Erdmann, Janeway, Keen, and O'Reilly disembark
5. July 5, P.M. Arrives at Gray Gables, President Cleveland's summer home on Buzzards Bay, near Bourne, Massachusetts

mollify them, Dan Lamont, reprising his role as the president's unofficial press secretary, issued a statement. He said the trip from New York to Gray Gables had been "leisurely." He said the presidential party had "cruised slowly through Long Island Sound and came to anchor when they found good fishing grounds." As for the president's health, Lamont said it was "excellent, excepting that he was suffering from a slight attack of rheumatism." The statement continued:

> The president has faithfully earned the brief rest which he hopes to have and he trusts that he will not be bothered by office-seekers while enjoying the comforts of his home. President Cleveland will have only about four weeks in which to rest and recuperate and

he desires to do so without annoyance. He must have perfect quiet before he returns to the Capital City and enters upon his arduous duties.

No one knows how hard the president has worked for the last four months, and the rest which he seeks in this admirable climate he hopes will not be denied him.

But a letter Dr. Bryant sent from Gray Gables to Dr. Keen in Philadelphia that same day tells a different story:

> We arrived at home in fine condition. At the present time, everything is as good as can be wished. I write to give you this information and also to thank you for your cooperation and support in the matter. I am convinced that my judgment regarding yourself was correctly made. Do not by word or intimation indicate the fact to anyone that you were with me, that is anyone other than your own family, and even they should not know whom you saw with me. The policy of the affair will be indicated by statements of friends to the public press.

That night, an intrepid reporter for United Press went to Gray Gables and managed to corner Dr. Bryant on the porch.

"Doctor," the unidentified reporter said, "a number of conflicting stories are told concerning the illness of the president. Some of them make the matter very serious. You would confer a great favor by making some sort of official statement."

"The president is all right," Bryant answered emphatically.

"From what is he suffering?"

"He is suffering from rheumatism, just as it was reported this afternoon. Those reports were correct."

"Then, doctor, the report that he is suffering from a malignant or cancerous growth in the mouth and that an operation was necessary and had been performed to relieve it is not correct?"

"He is suffering from the teeth, that is all."

"Has an operation been performed?"

"That is all," said Bryant, who ended the interview there.

On the morning of the next day, Friday, July 7, the interview was published verbatim in newspapers nationwide. Bryant's refusal to categorically deny that an operation had been performed on Cleveland only intensified speculation as to the president's health. The doctor summarily declared the interview a fake. Insisting he'd never even spoken with a United Press correspondent, Bryant issued a statement. "The president is absolutely free from cancer or malignant growth of any description," he said. "No operation has been performed, except that a bad tooth was extracted."

But it was too late. Sensing a stupendous story, newspapers large and small from Maine to Maryland immediately dispatched reporters to Gray Gables. Bryant was furious. He suspected the source of the cancer rumors was Ferdinand Hasbrouck, the dentist whose departure from the *Oneida* had been delayed. Bryant sent Hasbrouck his $250 fee by messenger. The two men never spoke again.

The indefatigable Dan Lamont was determined to stamp out the flames of speculation before they flared into a conflagration. He summoned the president's private secretary, Robert O'Brien, to Gray Gables to assist him. In the coming days, weeks, and months, Grover Cleveland's closest friends, advisers, doctors, and even his pregnant wife would all dissemble to perpetuate the myth that the president was well. With their help, Lamont would engineer a brazen and elaborate cover-up on behalf of a president whose reputation for honesty was unquestioned. It would be a spectacular example of what later generations would call damage control.

That same morning, July 7, Lamont invited Joseph Jefferson over to Gray Gables to call on the president. Jefferson, who was famous for his portrayal of Rip Van Winkle on stages around the world, afterward issued a statement in which he said he found the president "much improved in general health and very cheerful." It's doubtful the president was either. In fact, it's doubtful Jefferson even saw him at all. The purpose of the visit was not social; it was to prepare the way for the bigger lies to come.

Throughout the day, reporters continued to descend on Walker's, the small hotel down the road from Gray Gables. By the afternoon they numbered more than fifty. Lamont sent word that he would meet with them at seven o'clock that evening "with a full explanation of everything." Until then, he requested that they report nothing.

At the appointed hour, the reporters made their way along the dirt road to Gray Gables. Lamont was waiting for them in an old barn about two hundred yards from the house. Lamont didn't want prying eyes to see anything that might contradict the tale he was about to tell. As Robert O'Brien later wrote, "My personal impression at the time was that if ever one reporter got inside the house and detected the hospital odors and particularly if he caught sight of Mr. Cleveland who was beginning to sit up in a bathrobe the jig would be up—for he looked like a very sick man." Years later, O'Brien recalled the scene inside the barn that night:

> [Lamont] greeted the men cordially and with apparent frankness. He told them that it was really very foolish to make such a stir over a matter essentially trivial; that while the president suffered from an attack of rheumatism, to which he was occasionally subjected, the thing that had occasioned the prolonged journey on Mr. Benedict's yacht was only a bad case of dentistry. The president, besides being very busy, never enjoyed having a dentist work over him. In consequence he had allowed his dental work to fall so badly into arrears that he had finally felt compelled to go on the yacht; here he could be cool and comfortable and let the dentist make a thorough job of it. This had been done.

Lamont blamed the "opposition"—the silverites—for spreading false rumors about the president's health. Just that day, Lamont insisted, the president had played checkers with Mrs. Cleveland.

O'Brien said Lamont's strategy was simple: "Nothing but dentistry was the slogan." As Grant had done nine years earlier, Cleveland would dismiss his cancer as a toothache.

The reporters were skeptical, of course, and they peppered Lamont with questions. Who was the dentist? What was the exact nature of the dentistry? When, precisely, was the work performed? "These questions did not stump the resourceful Lamont," O'Brien wrote, "who dismissed them with the remark that they were too trivial to talk about." After deflecting a few more questions with a mix of charm and mock indignation, Lamont told the reporters he would not "dignify the subject by talking more about it" and ended the curious press conference.

As they trudged back to the hotel under the darkening summer sky, the reporters began debating heatedly among themselves. Half of them believed Lamont's story. The other half did not. On one point, however, there was unanimous agreement: they must all stand united and report the same story. This, according to O'Brien, was an arrangement that reporters often made. It was better for everyone to be on the same page—even if it was the wrong page. Which of the stories they would report would be decided once they got back to the hotel, perhaps over drinks.

Later that evening, Lamont sent a telegram to the secretary of state, Walter Gresham, who had heard the rumors about the president's health but knew nothing of his true condition. Lamont also made sure a copy was sent to the reporters at the hotel.

> Buzzards Bay, July 7, 1893
> To Walter Q. Gresham, Secretary of State:
> The President is laid up with rheumatism in his knee and foot, but will be out in a day or two. No occasion for any uneasiness.
>   D. S. LAMONT

And something else happened that night that threatened to blow the president's cover. At 7:20 that evening—the very moment Lamont was meeting with the reporters in the old barn at Gray Gables—Samuel Blatchford, a supreme court justice, passed away at his summer home in Newport, Rhode Island. Blatchford was seventy-three and had been in failing health for a year, so his death was hardly unexpected. For

Cleveland, however, the timing couldn't have been worse. The funeral would be held in four days in Newport, which was just fifty miles down the coast from Gray Gables. It would be impossible for the president to attend, of course. His absence would be most conspicuous, and it would certainly raise more troubling questions about his health.

Blatchford's passing also presented the beleaguered president with another momentous task: he would have to nominate the late justice's successor on the high court. It would take almost seven months for Cleveland to announce his choice: Louisiana senator Edward White. An ex-Confederate soldier, White would vote to uphold segregation in the notorious case of *Plessy v. Ferguson* in 1896. Fourteen years later, White was elevated to chief justice by President Taft.

<hr />

What did Vice President Adlai Stevenson make of all the rumors about the president's health? As previously noted, Cleveland hoped to hide everything from his would-be successor, whom he didn't trust. Stevenson

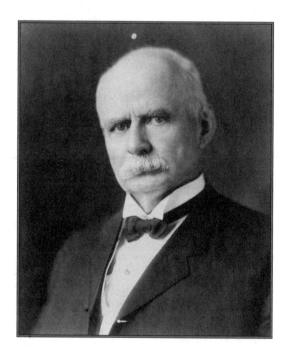

Vice President Adlai Stevenson opposed Cleveland's efforts to repeal the Silver Purchase Act. Before the 1940s, vice presidential nominees were usually chosen with little input from the candidate at the top of the ticket, often leading to uncomfortable arranged marriages. LIBRARY OF CONGRESS

was a silverite and opposed the president's efforts to repeal the Silver Purchase Act. Furthermore, Stevenson had surrounded himself with pro-silver advisers, whom Cleveland derisively dubbed the "Stevenson cabinet." For his part, Stevenson said Cleveland was "courteous at all times," but he admitted he was less an adviser to the president than "the neighbor to his counsels." Stevenson saw some humor in his awkward union with Grover. He liked to compare himself to James Buchanan's vice president, John Breckenridge, who told of being consulted by Buchanan just once—about the wording of a Thanksgiving proclamation.

Stevenson was attending the Fourth of July ceremonies at the World's Fair in Chicago when he learned of Cleveland's secretive and suspicious sojourn on the *Oneida*. It's safe to assume the vice president was reasonably curious about the president's health. In any event, he was determined to find out what was really going on. On July 6, he left Chicago, telling reporters he intended to go to Gray Gables to "consult with the president." He never made it. When Cleveland got wind of Stevenson's plan to visit him unbidden, the vice president was sent a telegram informing him that his counsel was neither necessary nor desired. Taking no chances, Cleveland ordered Stevenson to meet with Democratic Party leaders—on the West Coast. For the next month Stevenson would take a combination of trains, stagecoaches, and steamers from Washington to San Diego to Seattle and back to Washington.

At least Stevenson had fun. On the way home he rode the rails of the Great Northern, a brand-new line that ran from Seattle to St. Paul, and one of the few major railroads to avoid bankruptcy so far that year. "The marvelous switchback track in the Cascades and the grandeurs of Tumwater Canyon cannot be equaled in America," he told a reporter in St. Paul. "We enjoyed every moment of the trip, and could tell enough to fill columns of the wonders of the mighty Northwest."

After they returned from the barn at Gray Gables, the reporters convened at their hotel to decide which story they would file for the next day's papers. It was an animated discussion. A reporter for one of the more sensational New York dailies proposed a compromise: report the "malignant growth" story the following morning and the "dentistry" story a day later. He saw no harm in "throw[ing] a scare" into the country for twenty-four hours. But the more experienced scribes, many of whom knew Lamont well, were inclined to accept his version of events, and ultimately their point of view prevailed. The reporters unanimously agreed to report that the president was well. Grover Cleveland was given the benefit of the doubt—a benefit that modern presidents rarely enjoy.

Were the reporters naïve, or were they complicit in the cover-up? Perhaps a little of both. Grover's reputation for honesty made the whopper they were fed more palatable to the reporters. After all, hadn't he proven himself to be honest when he issued his famous dictum to "tell the truth" after the story of his illegitimate child broke in 1884? This was certainly an argument that swayed some reporters at the hotel that night. Others may have been swayed by patriotism. Even if the president was seriously ill, what good would come of reporting the news when the nation was in peril?

Of course, it's also possible that Dan Lamont pulled some strings to guarantee favorable coverage. Robert O'Brien believed "Lamont brought influence to bear upon the Associated Press to make it receptive to the conservative story which he [told] that night to the assembled journalists."

By whatever means, Lamont achieved his objective. On Saturday, July 8, exactly one week after the operation, the reporters at Gray Gables, without exception, filed stories reassuring anxious Americans that their president was just fine. "Mr. Cleveland Is Better," read the headline in the *New York Tribune*. "Likely to Recover in a Few Days."

"The President Is All Right," the *New York Times* chimed in. "Alarming Stories of His Illness Without Foundation." "The assertion that President Cleveland is seriously afflicted with any malady is all nonsense," the paper reported. His only affliction was "an ordinary, everyday sort of toothache," and "surely nothing more will be heard of [a] 'cancerous growth.'" The *Times* concluded, "Those who look for ominous news from Gray Gables just now will not get it."

In an editorial, the *New York World* chastised readers who had dared to question the paper's coverage of the president's alleged illness:

The persistent attempts to misrepresent and exaggerate President Cleveland's ailment are something more than scandalous at this time. If these reports were believed by the public they might very easily, and probably would, precipitate a financial panic. The *World* has had direct and unquestioned information from the first and has given the exact facts. It is a pity if a president cannot have 'a touch of rhoumatiz' [*sic*] and a toothache without giving rise to a swarm of rumors and false reports—some of them far more malignant than his disease.

George Babbitt, the influential editor of the *Boston Herald* wrote, "The buzzards will please keep aloof from Buzzards Bay."

On July 8, the same day many of these stories appeared, Attorney General Richard Olney went to Gray Gables to help the president prepare his message on the repeal of the Silver Purchase Act for the special session of Congress. Olney had been trying to get an appointment with Cleveland for two weeks without success. He knew nothing of the president's condition, and when he finally met with him at Gray Gables, he was shocked by what he saw:

[The president] had changed a great deal in appearance, lost a great deal of flesh, and his mouth was so stuffed with antiseptic wads that he could hardly articulate. The first utterance that I understood was something like this: "My God, Olney, they nearly killed me." He did not talk much, was very depressed, and at that time acted, and I believe he felt, as if he did not expect to recover.

Grover handed Olney what he had written so far. It amounted to just twenty or thirty lines. "He was very depressed about the progress he was making and complained that his mind would not work, and, upon my suggestion that I might perhaps be of assistance, was evidently much relieved." For the next two or three days, Olney stayed at Gray Gables, drafting a message that, he later claimed, "was approved by Mr. Cleveland practically as drawn."*

Olney found the visit very distressing. He was now the only member of the cabinet besides Lamont who really knew what was going on. He was, of course, sworn to secrecy, and required, like everybody else privy to that information, to prevaricate. After he met with the president, Olney told reporters that "Mr. Cleveland was doing finely, was in good spirits, and apparently enjoying excellent health, and that his illness was all confined to his knee and foot."

It was all balderdash. As Robert O'Brien revealed, the president was still bedridden as late as July 7. And according to Olney's account, Cleveland was not yet fitted with a prosthetic device on July 8, presumably because his wound was not sufficiently healed. The president could barely speak and most certainly couldn't eat solid foods. Olney's account also confirms that Cleveland, a notorious workaholic, was still virtually incapable of executing his official duties.

But Cleveland was blessed with a strong constitution and he recovered from the surgery with surprising swiftness. His kidney disease was not aggravated by the ether. He suffered no postoperative infections. Dr. Bryant was amazed by the rapidity with which his patient seemed to heal. On the afternoon of Monday, July 10, the president ventured out in public for the first time since the operation nine days earlier. Accompanied by Lamont and Bryant, he went fishing in his catboat, the *Ruth*. The party sailed about five miles down the bay and anchored off a small peninsula called Wings Neck. They spent several hours casting and were rewarded with a haul of scup, blackfish, and bass. As they were sailing for home, a boat filled with reporters caught up with them.

"What luck today?" one of the reporters shouted.

---

* Most Cleveland biographers believe Olney gave himself too much credit and that the final draft of the address was almost entirely the product of Grover's intellect, not his attorney general's.

"Fairly good," answered Lamont.

The president, of course, said nothing.

The *Ruth* docked at Gray Gables at four o'clock. Frances was waiting for her husband. "Mr. Cleveland," one correspondent noted, "jumped onto the landing wharf with considerable agility and walked up the pathway to Gray Gables without assistance."

The following day, Tuesday, July 11, Grover, again accompanied by Lamont and Bryant, rode a carriage into Bourne to pick up his mail at the town's post office. That afternoon, the three men went fishing again, this time staying out almost until sunset. It's likely that, by then, the president had been fitted with the prosthesis that allowed him to better enunciate. Kasson Gibson, the New York prosthodontist recruited by Bryant, had set up a makeshift dental laboratory in one of the rooms at Gray Gables. Gibson made a plaster cast of the hole inside the president's mouth and used the cast to fashion a vulcanized-rubber device known as an obturator, which plugged the hole. "The vulcanite plate," Gibson explained, "was made without teeth, gold clasping the cuspid tooth on the left, second bicuspid and molar on right, bridging across the opening, with a thick round edge where it came in contact with the cheek." The obturator was instrumental in maintaining the secret. As Dr. W. W. Keen later wrote, "This supported the cheek in its natural position and prevented it from falling in. When it was in place, the president's speech was excellent, even its quality not being altered." However, Robert O'Brien, Cleveland's private secretary, disagreed. "His voice was visibly affected in the opinion of those who heard him regularly," O'Brien wrote many years later. In any event, Gibson earned high praise from the one person who mattered most: the patient. After Gibson sent the president a new prosthesis in October, Grover responded with a letter of thanks:

My dear Doctor,

I hasten to announce that you have scored another dental victory and a greater one than has before attended your manipulation of my corpus.

The new plate came last night. I looked at it quite askance—in point of fact with disfavor. I put it in this morning. It is now about 11 o'clock at night. I have worn it all day with the utmost ease and comfort without a shred of packing of any kind. I took it out to cleanse it after breakfast and lunch, but found very little on or behind it, that needed attention. My wife says that my voice and articulation are much better than they have been for a number of days. I have not had the plate out since dinner.

I feel very well as you may suppose over my new machine. The double-header, as I call it—the one you built up and afterwards cut down—I cannot make work very well, but the new one promises to be such a comfort that I expect to get on nicely with it and the old stand-by you first made . . .

Yours very sincerely,
Grover Cleveland

By Thursday, July 13, Grover had practically resumed his normal routine at Gray Gables: fishing, visiting friends, entertaining guests, sitting on the porch to imbibe the fresh sea air. He was seen in public with ever-increasing frequency. His sister, Mary Hoyt, left for her home in Nebraska that day. Dan Lamont left Gray Gables for New York the next day. Likewise, the reporters who had flocked to Buzzards Bay the previous week also began drifting home. Whatever had been ailing him, the president was clearly recovering nicely.

And so the questions about Grover's health faded away. Even skeptics began to accept the assurances that he was in good health. "The president gained in strength rapidly enough to justify the most optimistic expectations of his physicians," wrote Robert O'Brien.

Dr. Bryant also planned to leave Gray Gables, but when he examined the president around July 15, he discovered something that made him nervous. As he later wrote, "A suspicious looking growth [had] appeared at the inner margin of the wound which it was deemed wise should be removed for the sake of giving the patient the benefit of every doubt." Bryant hastily reconvened the surgical team for a second operation on the *Oneida*. Drs. Erdmann, Janeway, Keen, and O'Reilly went to Elias Benedict's Greenwich home, where they boarded the yacht in privacy. It is noteworthy that Dr. Hasbrouck was not asked to participate. It is possible that the second operation was performed entirely with a local anesthetic, such as a cocaine solution, making Hasbrouck's expertise in general anesthesia unnecessary. But it's more likely that Bryant, suspecting Hasbrouck was the source of the cancer rumors that began spreading soon after the first operation, no longer considered the dentist trustworthy.

The *Oneida* sailed to Gray Gables, where the president and Dr. Bryant boarded on the morning of Monday, July 17. Before embarking, Grover bade Frances an "affectionate adieu," which, according to one report, caused "some of the wiseacres to predict that he is off for a long cruise." The president, it was reported, "appeared in the best of health and spirits." Reporters were informed that he was going on a fishing excursion for about two days.

That afternoon, while the *Oneida* cruised the waters of Buzzards Bay, Bryant "removed . . . the suspicious appearing tissue and re-cauterized the entire surface of the wound with the galvanocautery," Dr. Keen later wrote, adding, "This operation was brief and the president recovered quickly."

The doctors were put ashore at Newport the next night. The *Oneida* returned to Gray Gables the following day, July 19. Relaxing on the porch of the big gray house with Frances that evening, Grover appeared the picture of contentment and good health. The few reporters still covering the president never suspected a thing.

Still, Grover's recovery was far from complete. On July 23, Charles Hamlin, a young Treasury Department official who later became the first Federal Reserve chairman, paid Cleveland a visit. Hamlin went to Gray Gables to deliver some statistics on the money question that Grover had asked him to prepare. "President appeared not well at all," Hamlin wrote in his diary. "Had his mouth evidently packed with some kind of bandage—could not speak distinctly. Seemed to me to have some serious trouble with his mouth—looked thoroughly tired out."

However, Hamlin noted the president was at least well enough to have a "long talk" with him about the economy. Before leaving, Hamlin noted, he "saw also Mrs. C. and Ruth who gave me some flowers."

———————————— ❧ ————————————

While Cleveland was convalescing, the economy was not. On July 11, four more banks failed, including the Kansas City Safe Deposit and Trust Company, the largest savings bank in Missouri, and Thornton's Banking House, which had been regarded as one of the strongest and safest banks in central Illinois. The Thornton's failure left hundreds of farmers penniless. Two weeks later, the New York, Lake Erie and Western Railroad, better known simply as the Erie, went into receivership, sending stocks tumbling again. Under the deceptively bland headline "Trade Is Not Brisk," the *New York Times* on July 29 listed business closings and layoffs that had been announced the previous day:

> Six mills in Rhode Island closed
> A mill in Lowell, Massachusetts, reduced to half time
> A mill in Saco, Maine, closed
> A mill in Bridgeport, Connecticut, reduced to half time
> A factory in Wilmerding, Pennsylvania, cut wages by twenty
>   percent
> A steel mill in Pittsburgh closed, with 500 workers laid off
> A mill in Harrisburg closed, with 400 workers laid off
> A mill in Ishpeming, Michigan, closed, with 200 workers laid off
> Iron-ore mines in Tower and Ely, Minnesota, closed
> A coal mine in San Antonio closed, with "a large number of
>   men" laid off

And that was just one day. The panic had become, in the words of Henry Adams, a "financial storm . . . the most deep-seated and far-reaching in the history of the country." In South Carolina, farmers were unable to sell cotton, simply because the buyers had no money to pay for it. In the upper Midwest, the Pillsbury flour mill purchased wheat with scrip, the equivalent of IOUs. The production of consumer goods, including musical instruments, furniture, jewelry, and clocks, plummeted or ceased altogether. Sales of horse-drawn carriages would never recover from the Panic of 1893. By the time the economy finally improved, carriages had been supplanted by other forms of transportation, including urban mass transit and the automobile. Even distilleries were idled. "The entire trouble is that the people have no money to buy whiskey," a St. Louis wholesaler lamented. Most alarmingly, the output of food for domestic consumption fell by 3.1 percent from 1893 to 1894, meaning many families went hungry. Overall, economists have estimated that the American economy operated at 20 to 25 percent below capacity during the panic.

There were no reliable unemployment statistics, so it is impossible to know exactly how many people were jobless that summer. But estimates range as high as three million nationwide—an unemployment rate of perhaps 20 percent. To get a handle on the problem, Montana created a Bureau of Agriculture, Labor, and Industry in 1893, the first state bureau of its kind. Other states soon did likewise.

Whatever the number of unemployed, it was, in the words of Charles Dawes, a Nebraska lawyer and future vice president, "appalling."

To many, the growing number of gaunt tramps roaming the cities and countryside looking for work was alarming and frightening. In Kansas, Governor Lorenzo Lewelling ordered police to leave "law-abiding tramps" alone. But other states, including Maryland and Massachusetts, passed harsh new anti-vagrancy laws to crack down on the itinerant unemployed.

Some local governments tried to help the jobless. Boston paid unemployed men $1.25 a day to chop wood. Other cities followed suit. Public works projects were launched in Chicago, Cincinnati, New York, and St. Louis—the first major efforts at public works relief in a depression. But most government officials shared Grover's opinion that the "lessons of paternalism ought to be unlearned." The vast majority of relief efforts would be organized by private organizations, mainly churches and labor unions, which were strained to the breaking point by the task of caring for the numberless indigent.

With the special session on the Silver Purchase Act rapidly approaching, the goldbugs and the silverites girded for a battle that some believed would be more than metaphorical. Colorado's pro-silver governor, Davis H. Waite, told a rally in Denver that "it is better, infinitely better, that blood should flow to the horses' bridles rather than our national liberties should be destroyed." (This earned Waite the alliterative, if unflattering, nickname Bloody Bridles.) Waite threatened "another revolution" if the law was repealed.

A Congregational minister in Denver said any member of Congress from the West who voted for repeal "should not be shot when he returned home, but should be put into a tank of kerosene and fire set to him."

In Nevada a pro-silver group issued a statement accusing President Cleveland of using "intimidation and bribery and executive threats" to repeal the Silver Purchase Act. "The friends of silver . . . are energetically organizing for the conflict."

So, too, were the friends of gold, who pointed out that the United States Treasury had purchased $147 million worth of silver—more than a third of the world's output—since the law had passed, with no discernible economic benefit. Why buy more?

In an editorial entitled "What's the Matter with Kansas?," *Emporia Gazette* editor William Allen White mocked one silverite Kansan as a "shabby, wild-eyed, rattle-brained fanatic" and another as "an old human hoop skirt." To the goldbugs, the silverites were rabble—and dangerously radical rabble at that.

It is hard for us to imagine today just how provocative the money question was in 1893. It was as divisive and vexing as any of today's hot-button political issues—think gay rights and gun control. It permeated every nook and cranny of American culture, and, even more than a century later, the debate still reverberates, often in unexpected places.

In 1888, Lyman Frank Baum caught Western fever. Baum was a sales-
man from upstate New York who dreamed of striking it rich. So, like
tens of thousands of other adventurous Americans, he headed west.
Baum, his wife Maud, and their two children moved to Aberdeen, a
small town in the Dakota Territory, in what would become the state
of South Dakota the following year. He opened a general store called
Baum's Bazaar, where his customers, mostly farmers, bought everything on credit. But there was a terrible drought that year—and the
next—and the farmers were unable to pay their bills. The store went
bankrupt in 1890. Undeterred, Baum next tried his hand at journalism.
He took over a local newspaper called the *Aberdeen Saturday Pioneer*. The
work suited Baum, who seemed to have a natural gift for writing. He
enjoyed penning editorials, many of which had a decidedly liberal bent.
One called for women's suffrage, not a universally popular sentiment
in South Dakota, where women would not win the vote until 1918. In
another, nakedly racist, editorial, however, Baum called for the exter-
mination of Native Americans. As a newspaperman, Baum must have
followed the debate over the money question very closely.

The *Saturday Pioneer* proved enormously popular, but nobody in
Aberdeen could afford to buy it—even at just five cents a copy—much
less pay to advertise in it. The newspaper lasted barely more than a year
before it went bankrupt like Baum's Bazaar. Baum, by this time completely cured of Western fever, moved to Chicago, where he found a job
working for the *Evening Post*. He had lived just three years in Aberdeen,
but the experience left a deep impression on him, particularly the plight
of the drought-stricken and deeply indebted farmers.

In Chicago, L. Frank Baum began writing children's books in his
spare time, meeting with some success. In 1900 he published his most
famous: *The Wonderful Wizard of Oz*.

Many scholars believe the book is an allegory for the money question, with a decidedly pro-silver bent. In Baum's story, Dorothy wears
silver shoes, not ruby slippers, as in the movie version. The Yellow Brick

Road represents gold. Dorothy herself represents the archetypal American everyman. The Scarecrow is the farmer; the Tin Man, the Eastern capitalist greedy for oil; and the Cowardly Lion, a spineless politician. The good witches are from the North and the South. The wicked witches are from the East and the West. The word "Oz" itself can be interpreted as an abbreviation for ounces—as in gold and silver. Baum would always insist he'd written the story "solely to pleasure children," but Oz became such a lucrative franchise that the author had no interest in politicizing it. In any event, the parallels are striking. As historian Gretchen Ritter writes, "Baum lived in the midst of a highly charged political environment and . . . he borrowed from the cultural materials at hand as he wrote."

If Grover Cleveland was the inspiration for the Cowardly Lion, L. Frank Baum never said as much. Throughout his medical ordeal, however, the president had shown himself to be anything but a coward.

Even in his incapacitated state, Cleveland understood the political math involved in repealing the Silver Purchase Act. There were 356 seats in the House and 88 in the Senate, so he needed 179 votes in the lower chamber and 45 in the upper to win repeal. And although his party— the Democrats—controlled both chambers, party lines in this debate were irrelevant. It was, as always, a sectional issue. Representatives and senators from the East were inclined to support repeal, regardless of party affiliation. Those from the South and the West were not.

As he recuperated at Gray Gables, Grover pondered the possible outcomes. In his papers is a list showing where he believed members of the House stood on the issue. By his reckoning, 173 representatives were for repeal, 114 were opposed, and sixty-nine were undecided: close, but still not enough votes to guarantee repeal. In the Senate, where the pro-silver states were disproportionately represented, the vote would likely be much closer.

On the afternoon of Friday, August 4, Grover left Buzzards Bay to return to Washington for the first time since his operation. While he traveled in relative luxury, the trip was grueling. From Gray Gables he took a carriage to Woods Hole, a train to Newport, a ferry to New York, a carriage across town to a ferry to Jersey City, a train to Washington, and, finally, a carriage to the White House, arriving on the afternoon of the following day. The trip was the president's first conspicuous public appearance since the surgery, and at every stop his countenance was scrutinized for any sign of disease. On the whole, the verdict was positive. In Newport he was reported to be "looking well and not the least weary." In New York he appeared "well tanned" and "seemed to be in perfect health."

Two days later, on Monday, August 7, the special session convened. Congress received the president's message the next day. Rather than delivering it personally, however, Cleveland had the speech read by clerks in each chamber. Both audiences listened "in dead silence." Acknowledging that "distrust and fear [had] sprung up on every side," Cleveland blamed the "unfortunate financial plight" on "Congressional legislation touching the purchase and coinage of silver by the General Government." In other words: Congress, it's your fault. Now fix it.

Had he ever served in a legislative body, Cleveland might have been more tactful. But he hadn't, and the message harkened back to his days as Buffalo's blunt "veto mayor."

Yet the president's message wasn't completely intemperate: It did not even contain the inflammatory word "gold," and, beyond repealing the Silver Purchase Act, Cleveland only urged Congress, obliquely, to "put beyond all doubt . . . the intention and the ability of the Government to fulfill its pecuniary obligations in money universally recognized by all civilized countries."

Three days later, on August 11, a repeal bill was introduced in the House. And, on that same day, the president once again left the capital and returned to Gray Gables. Accompanied by Secretary Lamont, Grover slipped out of town on an early-morning train. As with his abrupt departure on June 30, his leaving was not discovered until he was already gone. The president left behind a statement explaining his sudden exodus, though it was not released until that afternoon.

I am going back to my summer home at the seashore because I am not sufficiently rested from the strain to which I have been subjected since the 4th of March to fit me again to assume the duties and labors which await me here. I have been counseled by those whose advice I cannot disregard that the further rest I contemplate is absolutely necessary to my health and strength. I shall remain away during the month of August, and shall devote myself to rest and outdoor recreation.

My day's doings will be devoid of interest to the public, and I shall be exceedingly pleased if I can be free from the attentions of newspaper correspondents.

That the president should abandon the capital on the brink of such an important debate was regarded as unusual and troubling. Many members of Congress were disappointed by the president's departure, especially when they learned he would not be making any appointments while he was away. Yet clearly the president was not well. The "strain" was too much.

The rumor mill—one of the few thriving industries left in the country—resumed full-scale production.

While Grover fished on Buzzards Bay, the House debated repeal. The debate was often tedious, but it was momentous, and the nation followed it assiduously. The papers reprinted speeches in their entirety. The arguments were already familiar by then, of course, so personality and passion tended to predominate. Both were embodied in silver's most eloquent defender in the House, a handsome thirty-three-year-old representative from Nebraska named William Jennings Bryan.

Born and raised in Illinois, Bryan had moved to Omaha to practice law in 1887. Three years later he was elected to Congress. He seized on the silver issue, and his silver tongue soon put him in the movement's vanguard.

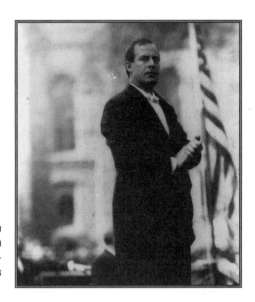

William Jennings Bryan, photographed in 1896. As a Democratic congressman from Nebraska, Bryan became a leader of the pro-silver movement. LIBRARY OF CONGRESS

When he rose to speak on the floor of the House on the afternoon of Wednesday, August 16, Bryan intended to read a speech he had labored for months to prepare. But as he looked around the chamber, with many of his colleagues drowsy in the heat, Bryan impulsively decided to forego his prepared address. He tossed the manuscript on his desk and began speaking extemporaneously. Almost immediately the languid representatives were roused by his impassioned plea for silver. He spoke with a special intensity, waving his left hand as if cracking an invisible whip. The battle was not between gold and silver, he insisted. It was between what we today would call the haves and the have-nots:

> On the one side stand the corporate interests of the United States, the moneyed interests, aggregated wealth and capital, imperious, arrogant, compassionless. . . . On the other side stand an unnumbered throng, those who gave to the Democratic Party a name and for whom it has assumed to speak. Work-worn and dust-begrimed, they make their mute appeal, and too often find their

cry for help beat in vain against the outer walls, while others, less
deserving, gain ready access to legislative halls.

Bryan held the chamber spellbound, and word of his oration spread
instantly throughout the Capitol and even the city itself. Senators were
drawn to the House chamber, and the public galleries filled. Though
he'd planned to speak for only an hour, Bryan went on to speak for
three, pausing only to sip a concoction of beef broth for refreshment.
When he finally concluded, exhausted, an unusually loud and long ova-
tion filled the chamber. Even a few goldbugs were moved to applaud.
Pro-silver representatives mobbed Bryan as if he'd just scored the winning goal in overtime.

Bryan's soaring rhetoric launched a political career that would last a
generation. He would become the unquestioned leader—the anti-Gro-
ver—of the pro-silver wing of the Democratic Party. But there would be
no come-from-behind victory for silver in the House. Bryan's eloquence
was not enough to save the Silver Purchase Act from repeal in the lower
chamber. The economy was too far gone. Something had to be done.
On his way to Washington for the special session, Ohio representative
Tom Johnson tried to cash a $200 check at a New York bank where he
was a large depositor. But the teller said he could only give the congressman fifty dollars. There was a money famine. After a conversation
with the bank's president, Johnson got his $200, but the experience left
him shaken. Johnson, a Democrat who had been undecided on repeal,
ended up voting in favor of it—as did nearly every other undecided
representative.

On August 28, after seventeen days of debate, the House voted in
favor of repeal by a margin of 239 to 108. The measure moved to the
Senate, where pro-silver senators were already threatening to filibuster.

Grover was still at Gray Gables when he got the news. "The action
of the House was wonderfully gratifying," he wrote, "and the majority
we secured was beyond our expectations."

It was a spectacular political victory, but his joy would be short lived,
for the very next day, August 29, the *Philadelphia Press* revealed what Grover had desperately fought to keep hidden: his cancer operation.

7

THE NEWSPAPERMAN

D R. CARLOS MACDONALD was not pleased when Dr. Ferdinand
Hasbrouck was late for his appointment in Greenwich on July 2,
1893. MacDonald had engaged Hasbrouck to administer anesthesia for
an important "last resort" operation. "I telegraphed to his office in New
York," MacDonald recalled, "and in reply was informed that his assis-
tants did not know where he was." After waiting more than an hour for
Hasbrouck to show up, MacDonald was forced to cancel the procedure
and send the patient home.

"The next day Dr. Hasbrouck appeared," MacDonald said. "He
found me in a very angry frame of mind but he asked me not to criticize
him until he had told his story." And what a story he told. Hasbrouck
said he had been unexpectedly and urgently summoned to assist in a
secret operation on President Cleveland and that the operation had been
performed on Elias Benedict's yacht, the *Oneida*. No less than a matter
of national security had prevented him from keeping his appointment.

Whether MacDonald was satisfied with Hasbrouck's explanation we
do not know. What we do know is that MacDonald repeated the story

to other doctors. One of the doctors to whom MacDonald told the story was Leander Jones, a prominent general practitioner in Greenwich.

And Jones just happened to be a good friend of an enterprising newspaperman named Elisha Jay Edwards.

He would write millions of words in his lifetime, but almost none about himself, so we know surprisingly little about Edwards. As a result, though he was one of the great reporters of his generation, he is little remembered today.

We do know that he was born in Norwich, Connecticut, in 1847, ten years after Grover Cleveland, with whom he had much in common. Both men were descended from famous preachers. One of Edwards's ancestors was Timothy Edwards, a minister whose son, Jonathan Edwards, was one of the great theologians of the eighteenth century. When he was sixteen, his family moved to New Haven. He graduated from Yale in 1870 and married Anna Scribner Jones, also descended from a prominent New England family, two years later. They would have three sons.

Edwards planned to pursue a career in law—again like Cleveland— and graduated from Yale's law school in 1873. He opened an office in New Haven, but shortly after he hung out his shingle, his career took a turn. He bought a stake in a small New Haven newspaper called the *Elm City Press* and soon became the paper's managing editor. Within months the paper's circulation rose from three hundred to nearly fifteen hundred copies daily. Edwards had long been interested in journalism. During law school he had worked for another New Haven paper, the *Palladium*. Evidently he found the newspaper business more appealing than the law. According to one account, Edwards discovered that journalism "offered a broader and more congenial scope for his endeavors." By 1874 he had sold his stake in the *Elm City Press* and become the managing editor of the *Norwich Bulletin*, a Republican paper. "Editing is evidently his forte," his Yale Law School yearbook noted, "uniting as he does liberality of thought with ability, being a gentleman at all times,

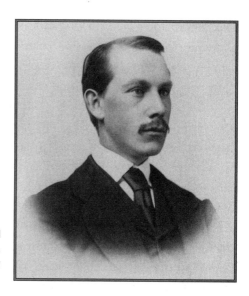

E. J. Edwards, photographed around
1870, the year he graduated from Yale.
MANUSCRIPTS AND ARCHIVES, YALE UNIVERSITY LIBRARY

and somewhat peculiar, perhaps, in allowing that there may be some honest men who do not agree with him politically."

His friends called him Eddie or Jay, but his byline read, "E. J. Edwards," the name by which he would be known professionally for the rest of his life. And although he had abandoned the law for good, E. J. Edwards put his legal training to good use in the newspaper business. He pursued stories with the tenacity of a prosecutor and the fairness of a judge. He was a gifted reporter, blessed with a photographic memory and a way with words. Somehow his work caught the discerning eye of Charles Anderson Dana, the formidable publisher of the mighty *New York Sun*, and in 1879 Dana hired Edwards.

It was an astonishingly lucky break for Edwards. As Allen Churchill points out in *Park Row*, his book about fin de siècle newspapers, the daydreams of most reporters at that time were largely devoted to envisioning being summoned to work for Charles Dana, who was one of the towering figures of nineteenth-century American journalism. Before the Civil War, Dana had worked as Horace Greeley's right-hand man at the *New York Tribune*, but he left that paper after the two men had a falling out. Dana then accepted a position in the Lincoln administration as a special observer on the western front of the war, where he befriended Ulysses S. Grant. Dana would champion Grant's presidential candidacy, but, consistent with his ostensible knack for making enemies, Dana became harshly critical of Grant once he was in office.

In 1868, Dana bought the *New York Sun* for $175,000. The paper had been founded in 1833 as a "penny paper," four densely typeset pages that sold for one cent. For a time it had been the daily newspaper with the highest circulation in the country, but after the war the *Sun* fell on hard times, a victim of increasing competition from other penny papers. By the time Dana bought it, the paper's daily circulation had dipped to forty-three thousand, far behind its New York competitors. Under Dana's brilliant tutelage, however, the *Sun* rebounded. By 1876 circulation had more than tripled to 131,000, and the newspaper was the most popular in the city. On November 8 of that year, in the heat of the disputed Hayes-Tilden presidential election, the *Sun* sold an astonishing 220,000 copies, a single-day sale that Dana claimed had never before been "equaled or approached."

The secret to Dana's success was simple and succinctly stated in one of the *Sun*'s promotional slogans: "Its news is the freshest, most interesting and sprightliest current, and no expense is spared to make it just what the great mass of the people want." Like other penny papers, the *Sun* carried its share of "sensation stories," what the newspaper historian Frank Luther Mott has defined as "the detailed . . . treatment of crimes, disasters, sex scandals, and monstrosities." But the *Sun* was also the first major newspaper to run what we now call human interest stories, articles that were provocative or amusing or intriguing but not necessarily newsworthy: a new variety of apple, the travails of a Chinese laundryman, the latest style in whiskers. One of the paper's editors coined the dictum, "If a man bites a dog, that's news."

What made these stories come alive was the writing—vivid and sparkling. Dana made sure of that. He was infatuated with the English language. As Allen Churchill puts it in *Park Row*, "The awesome man was fiendishly determined that every edition of the *Sun* stand as a monument to the ultimate in English." Reporters were known to be disciplined for grammatical errors in their copy. One was reportedly fired for using the word "balance" when, Dana believed, he should have used "remainder" instead. *Sun* stories were literate, poignant, whimsical. It was groundbreaking stuff. A good example of the paper's quirky style is the response that Francis Church, one of the *Sun*'s editorial writers, gave to an eight-year-old girl named Virginia O'Hanlon, who'd written a letter to the paper asking, "Is there a Santa Claus?"

"Yes, Virginia," Church replied on the *Sun*'s editorial page, "there is a Santa Claus."

Nominally the *Sun* was a Democratic paper, but Dana's mercurial temper and frequent feuds made it hard to tell. In any event, opinions were reserved for the editorial page, which was just as likely to contain an amusing essay as a condemnation of Dana's latest enemy. The *Sun* was at the forefront of the era's evolving journalistic standards. In most papers, objectivity took a backseat—if it took a seat at all—to entertainment and advocacy. It was not unusual for newspapers to simply invent "news" to sell papers. That's what the *Sun* had done before Dana took it over. In 1835 the paper published a series of articles describing life on the moon as discovered by an astronomer using a new "immense telescope." Among the inhabitants were giant walking beavers and winged humanoids. It was utter hogwash, but no matter: circulation skyrocketed.

Dana, however, wanted nothing to do with crude hoaxes. His *Sun* was a different paper, the proverbial newspaperman's newspaper. Dana had two rules for reporters: be interesting, and never be in a hurry. At a time when reporters had a reputation for being uncouth, ill-tempered, and intoxicated, Dana preferred to hire sober gentlemen, usually college graduates. (As a native of New Hampshire, Dana also had a special fondness for New Englanders like E. J. Edwards.) He paid his reporters a decent wage but made them work long hours: twelve-hour days were typical, and twenty-hour days were not unusual. And while he didn't hurry them, Dana did expect his reporters to be productive. In a typical week a reporter might turn out twenty-five thousand words, roughly one-third as many as are contained in this book. Dana was always on the lookout for new talent, and in 1879 he plucked E. J. Edwards from the journalistic obscurity of the *Norwich Bulletin* and dropped him into the most exalted newsroom in America.

We can imagine E. J. reporting for his first day of work at the *Sun*. He was thirty-two years old by then—not a youngster, certainly—though he still must have been nervous, perhaps even daunted by his new position. Through the crowded streets of the Lower East Side he made his way to a neighborhood near City Hall known as Newspaper Row. All the great papers were based there: the *Tribune*, whose nine-story building was the tallest in the city, the *Herald*, the *Times*, the *World*, the *Journal*, and, in a shabby six-story building on the corner of Nassau and Franklin, the *Sun*. Horse-drawn wagons jammed the streets. Scurrying among them were hundreds of newsboys, some as young as six, each eager to buy a bundle of one hundred penny papers hot off the presses for fifty cents. If a boy sold more than fifty papers, he would make a profit that day. If he sold fewer than fifty, he would lose money.*

Entering the *Sun* building, Edwards would have climbed a spiral iron staircase to the third floor, where the paper's newsroom was located. In this respect, too, the *Sun* was different: while reporters at other papers still worked in private offices, the *Sun*'s newsroom was open. Presiding over it from an office at the top of the staircase was the imperious Dana himself, stern and imposing in his full white beard.

The reporters worked at inclined tables illuminated by dim gaslights and, later, electric bulbs. They wrote their stories in longhand with pencils. They usually worked with their hats on, a tradition that prevented the theft of a precious beaver or derby by unscrupulous visitors—or colleagues. Edwards, like most young men of his time, wore a thick moustache. The older reporters sported full beards like Dana. Rare was the clean-shaven newspaperman.

Female reporters were not unheard of. An estimated two hundred women worked at New York newspapers in 1888. But the newsroom

---

* After the newsboys went on strike in 1899, the newspapers finally agreed to buy back their unsold copies.

was still an overwhelmingly male environment. The men dressed almost uniformly in white shirts with high, stiff collars and dark suits. Their clothing was fastened by laces or buttons; the zipper had not been invented yet. A few wore bow ties or ascots, but most wore neckties, which had only come into fashion after the war. On their feet they wore high leather shoes.

The newsroom was filled with smoke, though none from cigarettes. Only pipes and cigars were smoked in 1879, though a machine that could roll twelve thousand cigarettes an hour would be patented the following year, ushering in the golden era of the dread disease. The older reporters chewed tobacco, which they spit with impressive accuracy into brass spittoons strategically placed throughout the room. There was no clatter of typewriters, no ringing of telephones—only the din of shouted conversations and the unrelenting rumble of the presses in the basement, punctuated by urgent cries for a copyboy to deliver the latest dispatch to the typesetters and an occasional staccato burst of Morse code from a lone telegraph.

It was an exciting time to work in newspapers because, unlike today, America's appetite for them was practically insatiable. Between 1870 and 1890, the number of U.S. papers tripled from four thousand to twelve thousand. "The American newspaper press became a great turgid flood," writes Frank Luther Mott, "carrying over the whole land its popular education, its millions of words of information about matters important and trivial, its stimulation of commerce through advertising." That growth was fueled by huge technological advances in papermaking and printing. Allegedly inspired by observing wasps building their nests out of tree fibers, a German inventor named Friedrich Gottlob Keller devised a method for manufacturing newsprint out of cheap wood pulp instead of cotton fibers. This reduced the cost of newsprint by 75 percent between 1872 and 1892. Unfortunately it also reduced the durability of the paper. Newspapers printed on pulp deteriorate much more quickly than papers printed on fiber-based papers.

Simultaneously, the American mechanic Richard Hoe was perfecting a printing press that used a rotating cylinder, replacing the old flatbed press that had been in favor since Gutenberg. In 1847 Hoe received a patent on a "lightning press" capable of printing eight thousand pages per hour. By 1889 his company had developed a press that could print an astounding five hundred thousand pages per hour. These advances vastly reduced the cost of newspapers, for the first time making them widely available to the masses, who were increasingly able to read them: between 1870 and 1890, the U.S. illiteracy rate fell from 20 to 13.3 percent.

News gathering was rapidly changing, too. In the 1840s some news-papers used carrier pigeons to transmit news. The *Sun* even kept a pigeon coop on the roof of its building. A decade later came Morse's telegraph and then, in the 1870s, Bell's telephone. In the 1880s the clat-ter of typewriters began to be heard in newsrooms. The AP began using the machines in 1885. "A few years ago type writer copy was the excep-tion," a trade journal called the *Journalist* said in 1886. "Now it is the rule among the better class of journalists."

Many of the old guard, however, could never bring themselves to adopt the newfangled machine. Like many of his generation, E. J. Edwards would continue to write his stories out in longhand. But he was no reactionary. Edwards was an early adopter of the then revolutionary "interview technique" whereby reporters actually asked the subjects of their stories questions. This was controversial because, as newspaper historian Frank Luther Mott writes, the "questions were often flippant and the replies ill considered." The *Nation* said interviewing made "fools of great men." But the technique would prove enduring.

The explosive growth of newspapers resulted in fierce competition for readers, especially in the larger cities, and in 1883, just four years after Edwards joined the *Sun*, the paper faced a challenge to its suprem-acy in New York. Joseph Pulitzer, a thirty-six-year-old Hungarian immi-grant, bought the *New York World* and set his sights squarely on the *Sun*. Pulitzer had already enjoyed phenomenal success in St. Louis, where he'd bought the *Dispatch* at a sheriff's sale in 1878 and soon merged it with another paper, the *Post*. Under Pulitzer's management, the *Post-Dispatch* soon became the highest-circulated evening paper in the city.

But St. Louis could not contain his ambitions, and he set his sights on New York.

The *World's* circulation was twenty thousand when Pulitzer bought the paper. Sixteen months later it was one hundred thousand. Pulitzer's recipe for success was simple: appeal to the masses. At the time, some 80 percent of New York City's residents were either immigrants or the children of immigrants, and Pulitzer aimed the *World* directly at them. The stories were written so simply that even readers with limited English skills could understand and enjoy them. To paraphrase one Pulitzer biographer, other papers wrote about these people, but the *World* wrote for them.

But Pulitzer had other tricks up his sleeve. The *World* put a special emphasis on the sensational, especially crime. One critic said the *World* more closely resembled the *Police Gazette* than a daily newspaper. Pulitzer masterminded frequent publicity stunts and crusades, as when the *World* organized a campaign to raise money for the Statue of Liberty's pedestal after Congress failed to appropriate the necessary funds. More than 120,000 readers contributed sums as small as five cents to raise the $100,000 needed to erect the statue. Pulitzer also pioneered the use of illustrations, including pungent political cartoons. It was a style that would be widely replicated. It came to be known as yellow journalism, the name supposedly derived from a popular cartoon character called the Yellow Kid.

Dana's *Sun* and Pulitzer's *World* were running neck and neck in circulation when the 1884 presidential campaign rolled around. Dana still harbored a grudge against Cleveland for refusing to hire his friend, and the *Sun* editorialized bitterly against him. Dana said Cleveland had a "plodding mind, limited knowledge and narrow capacities." After the Maria Halpin story broke, Dana wrote, "We do not believe that the American people will knowingly elect to the Presidency a coarse debauchee who would bring his harlots with him to Washington and hire lodgings for them convenient to the White House."

Pulitzer, on the other hand, sensed Cleveland's popular appeal, especially among the working class, and he promoted his candidacy unrelentingly. The *World* listed four reasons for endorsing Cleveland: "1. He is an honest man; 2. He is an honest man; 3. He is an honest man; 4. He is an honest man." (Once Cleveland was elected, however, Pulitzer turned on him for refusing to appoint one of Pulitzer's friends to a post in Berlin.)

Meanwhile, Dana's vituperative attacks on Cleveland backfired. Rather than antipathy, they aroused sympathy for the candidate, and they certainly did the *Sun* no good. Alienated readers abandoned the paper in droves. During the campaign the *Sun*'s circulation nosedived from 137,000 to 85,000.

By Election Day the *Sun* had been eclipsed by the *World*.

In 1880, after just one year at the *Sun*, E. J. Edwards was named the paper's Washington correspondent. It was a major promotion, and in his new position Edwards thrived. In 1881 his coverage of the Garfield assassination earned high praise from Charles Dana himself, who called it, with typical brevity, "the best."

In Washington, Edwards also earned a reputation for dogged investigative reporting—at a time when such reporting was almost unheard of. In 1881 he helped uncover massive fraud in the Post Office Department. Edwards discovered that postal officials were accepting bribes in exchange for awarding contracts for mail delivery routes known as star routes. A Republican senator and an assistant postmaster general were implicated in the scheme, which cost taxpayers some $4 million (about $80 million in today's money). Though neither was convicted, the revelations contained in Edwards's reports ignited public fury and helped lead to the passage of the Pendleton Act, which reformed the civil service. The postmaster general at the time, Thomas James, later praised Edwards's work. "I cheerfully bear witness to the energy and zeal with which he entered into the great Star Route fight . . . and the vigorous manner in which he denounced the corrupt and defiant gang and held up their crimes to an indignant people."

In March 1887, Charles Dana opened a new front in his battle against Joseph Pulitzer's *World*. Dana launched an evening edition of the

Sun, and he summoned E. J. Edwards from Washington to be the new paper's managing editor. (Seven months later Pulitzer would retaliate by starting an evening edition of the *World*.) Back in New York, Edwards worked with a *Sun* reporter named Jacob Riis. Like Edwards, Riis was a newspaperman with a crusading streak, and the two shared an enthusiasm for investigative reporting. In 1888 the *Sun* published a series of articles by Riis detailing the deplorable living conditions in New York's tenements. The articles would later be published as a book entitled *How the Other Half Lives*. It is likely that Edwards helped Riis write the exposé. Edwards and Riis were pioneers in a genre that Teddy Roosevelt would label "muckraking," because the reporters dug up dirt. (Roosevelt once called Riis "New York's most useful citizen.") Their goal was not merely to expose the wicked or afflicted, nor was it sensationalism for its own sake. They saw their work as a public service, to educate readers, not merely to titillate them. Over the next twenty years, a parade of muckrakers would follow—Upton Sinclair, Lincoln Steffens, Ida Tarbell—ushering in the era of modern journalism.

Under Edwards's tutelage, the *Evening Sun* was an immediate success. "New York at last saw a modern, lively, well-edited, cheap evening paper," wrote one newspaper historian. Besides Jacob Riis, Edwards also worked with Richard Harding Davis, later a noted war correspondent and novelist. (Davis's father was L. Clarke Davis—one of Grover Cleveland's friends.) The *Evening Journal* restored some of Charles Dana's lost luster (and lucre), and the bearded curmudgeon was effusive in his praise of Edwards: "Mr. Edwards, in whatever responsibility he had been tested, excelled. As a reporter his work is beyond criticism. As an editorial writer he is pungent and thoughtful . . . and as an executive manager his career has been brilliant."

In 1889, after ten years at the *Sun*, Edwards left the paper for the *Philadelphia Press*. The *Press* was founded by John Forney in 1857 as a Democratic newspaper, but Forney abandoned the Democrats for the Republicans at the outbreak of the Civil War. Throughout the war, the *Press* was considered the foremost Republican paper in Pennsylvania, and thousands of copies of its weekly edition were distributed to Union

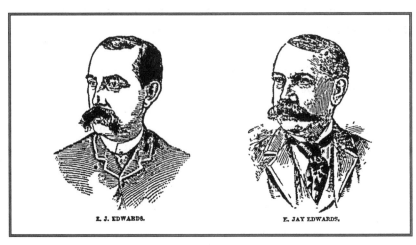

E. J. EDWARDS.   E. JAY EDWARDS.

These woodcuts of E. J. Edwards are from the 1890s, when he established himself as one of the first investigative reporters in American journalism. LIBRARY OF CONGRESS

soldiers. It was said that Forney supported Lincoln more fully than any other newspaper editor, though his editorials were remarkable for their courtesy and lack of invective. In 1880, Charles Emory Smith bought the paper. Like his predecessor, Smith was a devout Republican. He served as Benjamin Harrison's ambassador to Russia from 1890 to 1892 and would later hold positions in the McKinley and Theodore Roosevelt administrations. It was said that Smith hired only Union Army veterans to work in the paper's pressroom.

It was Smith who convinced Edwards to abandon the *Sun* for the *Press*. It probably helped that Smith, like Edwards, was a native of Connecticut. But more important to Edwards was the job: he would be the *Press*'s New York correspondent. It was a plum assignment. Working alone out of an office in the brand-new Schermerhorn Building on the Lower East Side, Edwards was given carte blanche to write about anything that suited his many fancies. Still composing in longhand, he filed a twenty-five-hundred-word column six days a week under the pen name Holland. The inspiration for this nom de plume is lost to history. Perhaps it was a nod to his new office: the New York Schermerhorns traced their roots back to a small Dutch village called Schermerhorn. His columns, which he called letters, touched on every imaginable issue, but Edwards especially enjoyed uncovering corruption in politics and business. Though well connected, he was never afraid to take on the rich and powerful. He also covered the arts and was not averse to including a bit of gossip as well. His columns would eventually be syndicated in several papers, including the *Cincinnati Enquirer* and the *Chicago Inter-Ocean*.

Holland's letters in the *Press* were notable for their lack of sensationalism. At the time, reporters like E. J. Edwards—scrupulous and intrepid—were still rare. As a columnist he quickly earned a reputation for honesty and fairness, and in newsrooms around the country a daily question was, "What does Holland say today?"

In 1892, Edwards met a struggling young writer so desperately poor he didn't even have a place to sleep. The writer's name was Stephen Crane, and he had recently been fired by the *New York Herald* for writing a sarcastic account of a labor union parade in which he described the marchers as "uncouth." Edwards lived in Greenwich, Connecticut, but he also kept an apartment on West Twenty-Seventh Street in Manhattan and let Crane crash there occasionally. Like Jacob Riis, Crane was fascinated by tenement life, and that fall he showed Edwards a manuscript he was working on. Called *Maggie: A Girl of the Streets*, the grim novel told the story of the title character, a prostitute unable to escape her tenement life. The following March, Crane showed Edwards another work in progress, a Civil War novel called *The Red Badge of Courage*. Edwards was deeply impressed by Crane's gritty writing, now recognized as an early example of naturalism in American literature. Crane's characters were tragic figures trapped in circumstances they could not escape.

Edwards must have been stunned and even humbled by the twenty-one-year-old Crane's work. Edwards convinced his editors at the *Press* to run a serialized version of *Red Badge*, which, Edwards later reported in his column, resulted in Crane receiving "a very flattering offer from one of the largest publishing houses . . . for a contract for the publication of that story in book form."* Edwards predicted that Crane would "become one of the great men of American letters." And indeed he would, partly due to Edwards's patronage. The publication of *Red Badge* in 1895 rocketed Crane to literary fame. But his career was fleeting. Just five years later, Crane died of tuberculosis at twenty-eight.

In 1893, in conjunction with the World's Fair in Chicago, the American Press Association, a newspaper syndicate based in New York, commissioned seventy-four experts in various fields to write columns predicting what their fields would look like one hundred years hence. E. J. Edwards was chosen to speculate on the future of journalism, and what he predicted reveals something about his belief in the powers of technology and science. In his essay, Edwards spoke with uncanny prescience:

> It is quite within the bounds of possibility that, by the year 1993, the mechanical work of publishing newspapers may be done entirely by electricity. The distributing of the printed papers also may be accomplished with such celerity as to vastly extend the legitimate field of any given journal.
>
> It is quite possible that, by the agency of forces just beginning to be understood, the reporter and editor will no longer be compelled to write. Rather, the spoken word may appear imprisoned in cold type . . . ,
>
> But the newspaper of 1993 must be as is the newspaper of today—nothing but the story of human achievement, and the story of human nature, and the story of the happenings of earth.

In 1893, E. J. Edwards was at the pinnacle of his career. His column was one of the most respected and widely read in the country. In Stephen Crane, he had discovered and nurtured a magnificent young talent. Even his predictions for the future were in demand. Yet a chance meeting that summer would alter the course of his career and eventually cost him his good reputation.

---

* Later accounts say the offer was perhaps less flattering than Crane had led Edwards to believe: no advance and a 10 percent royalty.

8

EXPOSED

L IKE THE REST of the country, E. J. Edwards had no inkling of Gro-ver Cleveland's illness when the president left Washington for his secret operation. Edwards blindly accepted Grover's explanation that he was merely going on holiday. On July 1, 1893, the day the president had much of his upper jaw removed on the *Oneida*, Edwards filed a long, breezy dispatch filled with gossip from New York. "[Interior Secretary Hoke Smith] is the only member of the cabinet who has dared to assert himself in the presence of the president. . . . [A] delegation of starv-ing miners may be sent to Washington from Colorado and Montana demanding from President Cleveland not bread but silver, which is the same thing to them." Toward the end of the column, Edwards noted that Elias Benedict was looking forward to spending the month with the president on Buzzards Bay. "Mr. Benedict says that Mr. Cleveland is as impatient for the sea bass fishing and as hungry for a day's sport trolling for bluefish as a schoolboy is for the first day of his vacation."

Then, one hot afternoon in late August, Edwards was returning to his Greenwich home after a brief vacation, when an old friend named Leander Jones flagged down his carriage. Jones was a well-connected doctor who counted among his patients some of the most powerful and wealthy figures of the Gilded Age, including Elias Benedict.

"I stopped," Edwards later wrote, "and he suggested that we go to one side for he had important news to tell me."

Jones said to Edwards, "We have narrowly escaped, I think, having Vice President Stevenson transferred from the Senate Chamber to the White House, as president."

Jones then proceeded to tell Edwards a most incredible story. He had learned from his friend and fellow doctor, Carlos MacDonald, that Grover Cleveland was ill. MacDonald had heard the story from a dentist named Ferdinand Hasbrouck, who said he'd taken part in an operation to remove a cancerous tumor from the president's mouth. The operation had been performed in total secrecy on the *Oneida*, Elias Benedict's yacht.

"Dr. Jones told me that the fact was sure to get out," Edwards later recalled, "and that he thought there was no reason why he should not tell me the story."

Edwards was stunned. He'd just been handed the scoop of the century, though in time he might wish he hadn't been. The story Jones told wasn't merely sensational, it was inflammatory, and Edwards understood the repercussions of reporting it. The White House still insisted the president had suffered from nothing worse than a toothache and a touch of rheumatism. By revealing that Cleveland had actually had a cancerous tumor removed from his mouth, Edwards would singlehandedly plunge the administration—and, perhaps, the country—into turmoil. He would also be risking his good name, for the president's allies were sure to kill the messenger, at least metaphorically.

Determined to confirm the story, Edwards went into the city early the next day to call on Ferdinand Hasbrouck, the dentist who'd told Jones's friend about the surgery in the first place. Hasbrouck lived in a handsome brownstone on 126th Street in Harlem, then the most fashionable neighborhood in the city. Edwards climbed the steps and rang the bell. Hasbrouck answered in his nightshirt. Edwards apologized for waking the dentist but explained that he was a newspaperman on deadline and needed to verify a few facts for a story he was writing. His introduction sounded innocuous enough. Hasbrouck invited Edwards inside.

Edwards waited in the parlor while Hasbrouck went upstairs to change into his morning coat. When he returned, the dentist took a seat close to Edwards. Hasbrouck was fifty, wiry, and handsome, with thinning dark hair and a full beard. He'd fought in the Civil War and was slightly deaf, apparently as a result of his battlefield experience. He cupped his hand behind his ear as Edwards spoke. Almost nonchalantly, Edwards told Hasbrouck everything he'd learned about the operation from Jones: the rendezvous on the *Oneida*, the makeshift operating theater below deck, the surgery itself.

Hasbrouck was flabbergasted. He listened in amazement.

"Some of the physicians who were aboard the yacht must have told you that story," he exclaimed. "You could not have obtained it in any other way!"

Edwards calmly asked Hasbrouck if the story was true.

Yes, Hasbrouck admitted, it was true. There was no point in denying it any longer. Hasbrouck told him everything. He also assured Edwards that the president had weathered the ordeal remarkably well and that the doctors were confident of his full recovery.

When the dentist finished, Edwards thanked him for his time and excused himself. He hurried to his office in the Schermerhorn Building and prepared a story about the operation for the *Press*, writing furiously in longhand as usual. He could not risk transmitting the story to Philadelphia by telegraph, however; a Western Union operator could not be trusted with such sensitive information. So Edwards phoned it in: he read the story to his editor at the *Press* over a telephone line. All the while, Edwards feared another reporter would beat him to the punch. "I was sure that the news would speedily get out," Edwards remembered, "and I had the newspaperman's desire to be the first to publish important news—what we call a 'beat.'"

It wasn't just a beat. It was one of the greatest scoops in the history of American journalism, and it is still the most detailed account of a medical procedure on a sitting president to be published without authorization.

The story appeared on the front page of the *Philadelphia Press* on August 29, 1893—the day after the House voted to repeal the Silver Purchase Act. In an age when exaggeration and even fabrication were acceptable journalistic devices, Edwards's account is notable for its absence of hyperbole. The prose is simple, restrained, sober—a little flowery sometimes, but never sensational or maudlin. Edwards forsook hysteria for accuracy.

In spite of its importance, though, Edwards's dispatch was not published underneath a banner headline. The bold, bellowing, page-wide headers that would come to epitomize yellow journalism were not yet in vogue in 1893. A few papers were experimenting with banners, usually to promote Sunday features or state editorial opinions. But the barriers that had long separated the eight narrow columns on every paper's front page would not be fully breached until 1894, when New York papers began using banner headlines for news stories. Banners quickly became standard, reaching their apogee during the Spanish-American War, when some headlines were so big they were only four or five characters wide.

But in 1893, newspapers were still adhering to the old "tombstone" style of stacking headlines within a single column over each story, so, at first glance, Edwards's scoop appears no more dramatic than any other story on the front page. Upon closer inspection, though, its magnitude is obvious:

THE PRESIDENT A VERY SICK MAN.
An Operation Performed on Him on Mr. Benedict's Yacht.
PART OF THE JAW REMOVED.

The story beneath these headlines takes up nearly three full columns on the front page. Edwards, writing under his usual penname of

PHILADELPHIA, TUESDAY MORNING,

THE PRESIDENT A VERY SICK MAN.

An Operation Performed on Him on Mr. Benedict's Yacht.

PART OF THE JAW REMOVED.

A Disease Whose Symptoms Gave Indications that It Might Be Sarcoma.

Mr. Cleveland's Present Condition Such as to Give Encouragement.

THE CASE NOT UNLIKE GRANT'S.

Four Days in Bed After the Use of Gas and Knife—Several of New York's Expert Physicians Concerned. Lamont's Devotion—The Several Causes.

From the Regular Correspondent of THE PRESS.

NEW YORK, Aug. 28.—Mr. Cleveland returns to Washington some day this week if all goes well and there are unusual reasons why, when he is again in the Capital, he should receive most tender, considerate and gentle sympathy and support, not only from those who are in public life, but also from the people themselves. He takes back to Washington a burden and a dread which he might very justly regard of greater moment than the financial situation which he has requested Congress instantly to ameliorate.

It is useless longer to conceal the fact that Mr. Cleveland is a sick man, perhaps a very sick man, and that the physicians have fear that mortal disease is lurking in his system, notwithstanding heroic efforts of surgery to remove it during the Summer. Secretary Lamont, who was here last week and whose anxiety was impressive and pitiful for his friends to see, said with something of the tone of sadness in his voice that there would be and could be no attempt on the part of the Administration to make any interference in the local politics of New York, and when asked why this was so, Lamont replied, saying it to Colonel

he concealed his suffering from his family, and it is probable that no one, excepting Secretary Lamont, knew that he had physical torture as well as mental anxiety to contend with. The pain did not yield to local and usual treatment. When the first careful examination was made, or when the suspicion was created that this trouble was due to no exposure of a dental nerve or to any usual disease of the teeth, my informants do not know; they do know that there was a time, shortly before the President issued his call for the extraordinary session of Congress, when it was determined that an operation was inevitable, how grave or extensive could not at first be determined. There were many things to consider—the family, the condition of the country, the determination to call Congress into extraordinary session and the necessity as it seemed for preserving professional confidences and therefore silence respecting this physical condition of the President.

It is probable that the decision to perform the operation while the President was upon Mr. Benedict's yacht was due to several reasons—one, perhaps, that the family, being in ignorance, might not be overwhelmed by anxiety and suspense; another, that if the operation was performed with surgical success the country might not be alarmed, since it was only too well understood that the ablest business men of both parties looked with confidence upon Mr. Cleveland, rather than his party, and contemplated any contingency by which the succession would revert to another with utmost anxiety.

THE OPERATION.

Mr. Cleveland, with Mr. Lamont, whose faithful attendance to one whom he respects as President, but regards with another and a more delightful sentiment, which approaches that of filial affection and has been a matter of much comment during the Summer, left Washington quite suddenly upon the day when the call for the extraordinary session of Congress was issued. Arrangements were made in this city with celerity, and Mr. Cleveland was met when he arrived here by Dr. Bryant and another physician, and by Dr. Hasbrouck, all of whom boarded the yacht with him. The baggage of these physicians contained the instruments of surgery and the apparatus for anaesthetic administration.

Dr. Hasbrouck had this latter apparatus in charge. He is a physician here who is regarded as being the most expert in the city in the administration of anaesthetic gas. He is employed professionally by most of the ablest physicians when it is deemed advisable to use gas rather than ether. Dr. Hasbrouck had been informed that the operation which called for his professional services might be a prolonged

Therefore Dr. Hasbrouck was kept upon the yacht two days, so that he might be at hand with his gas apparatus in case further operation should be necessary.

It gave the physicians great hope and encouragement that no such treatment was demanded. The wound seemed to heal easily, naturally, and that of itself furnishes considerable hope that the disease which called for this heroic treatment may after all not be malignant as was feared, but of that nature which the physicians call benign. It is the truth to say that there were suspicions that the disease might be of that malignant type which is called sarcoma, another form of the same disease which brought General Grant, with beautiful pathos, to his deathbed. There is now encouragement that it may not be that trouble, that the complaint, whatever it is, is not beyond the power of surgical science to control.

Mr. Cleveland recovered from the shock even better than the physicians had dared to hope he would. He was kept in bed, so treated that he slept much of the time, and after four days' absence, during which time the country was wondering where he was, it was deemed safe and advisable to permit him to land at Gray Gables. Those who were there knew that he was weak, that he had been suffering, but with a few exceptions it was supposed that his illness was due entirely to his rheumatic troubles.

The treatment indicated was absolute rest and such mental diversion as Mr. Cleveland's favorite recreation, fishing, afforded. His physician encouraged him to make these fishing trips, there being nothing else to do than to dress the wound, which seemed, after a few days, to be healing in a most satisfactory manner. It became necessary, however, for the President to return to Washington, and that journey and the necessity of living in Washington during the heated spell gave Mr. Cleveland's physician very great anxiety. It was, of course, noticed that Dr. Bryant was constantly at Gray Gables, accompanied Mr. Cleveland on his journey to Washington, and was with him much of the time there.

The doctor's practiced eye saw that there was danger—perhaps not of a recurrence of the disease, but of a setback in the process of healing—if the President remained in Washington, and his imperative command was that it was a higher duty for Mr. Cleveland, both to the country and to himself and family, to return immediately to Buzzard's Bay, the tonic air of which admirably agreed with him and served the more rapidly to overcome the effects of the operation.

It has been said that the extraordinary and unexplained departure of Mr. Cleveland from Wabington was not the act of a President who realized the desperate situation of the country; but Mr. Cleveland did realize it. He almost rebelled at the command of his physician. He knew his de-

---

E. J. Edwards's scoop about the secret operation on Grover Cleveland appeared on the front page of the *Philadelphia Press* on August 29, 1893. FREE LIBRARY OF PHILADELPHIA

Holland, begins with a paragraph casting Cleveland in a sympathetic light before making his startling revelation:

NEW YORK, Aug. 28.—Mr. Cleveland returns to Washington some day this week if all goes well and there are unusual reasons why, when he is again in the Capital, he should receive most tender, considerate and gentle sympathy and support, not only from those who are in public life, but also from the people themselves. He takes back to Washington a burden and a dread which he might very justly regard of greater moment than the financial situation which he has requested Congress instantly to ameliorate.

It is useless longer to conceal the fact that Mr. Cleveland is a sick man, perhaps a very sick man, and that the physicians have fear that mortal disease is lurking in his system, notwithstanding heroic efforts of surgery to remove it during the Summer. . . . The news which is here reported for the first time has been received from those whose sources of information are so accurate as to justify, even to compel, its publication.

Edwards describes Cleveland's ailment obliquely. Adhering to Gilded Age convention, he tiptoes around the word "cancer," instead referring to the disease as "that dread and mysterious enemy which physicians scarcely dare to name." He also writes that the disease might be "another form of the same disease which brought General Grant, with beautiful pathos, to his deathbed." The comparison to Grant, whose slow and painful death eight years before was still vivid in the public memory, must have perturbed Cleveland deeply.

Edwards also explains why Cleveland wanted to keep the operation secret: to keep the country from being "alarmed" and to keep his family from being "overwhelmed by anxiety and suspense." Like many others, Edwards was apparently under the misapprehension that Grover had concealed his condition even from his wife.

The operation itself is described only briefly:

When the time came the President of the United States submitted
himself to the surgeon as calmly, as gently, and as willingly as
though he were merely lying down for brief slumber. . . . The
operation did not require very long, but it entailed the cutting away
of a considerable part of the upper jaw bone upon one side, the
instrument boring through the bone and tissue as far as the orbital
plate.

Throughout the story, Edwards makes every effort to portray the
president as honorable, even heroic, at one point describing him as
"tormented by pain." He is also careful to reassure readers that the
president is no longer in any immediate danger. "The wound seemed to
heal easily, naturally, and that of itself furnishes considerable hope that
the disease . . . may after all not be malignant as was feared, but of that
nature which the physicians call benign." His tone is respectful—almost
reverential. Although Edwards was a Republican, he clearly admired
Cleveland, whom he once called "a man of extraordinary personal
force." It's virtually certain that the two men had met at some point,
since Edwards covered the 1884 presidential campaign for the *Sun* and
then served as the paper's Washington correspondent for the first two
years of Cleveland's first term.

In the article, Edwards also addresses the assertion that the president had merely had some dental work performed on the *Oneida*, and
he anticipates the denials that will inevitably issue from the Executive
Mansion:

The physicians believe that they have removed all of the diseased
tissue and bone. . . . Of course in doing this teeth were extracted,
so that the physicians were truthful when they afterward said
that the President had had some teeth pulled out while he was
on Mr. Benedict's yacht. They were also well within the rules of
professional diplomacy when they denied that any other operation
than that of ordinary gentle surgery had been performed, and they

now defend these statements and are quite likely publicly to insist
that they said all that was necessary to say, or that the operation
justified when they announced that Mr. Cleveland had merely had
some teeth extracted.

Edwards's story was certainly spectacular, but, since it was based
almost exclusively on Hasbrouck's recollection of events, it was not
complete. Of the six doctors present at the operation, Edwards iden-
tifies just two in his article: Hasbrouck and Bryant. He also suggests
that Cleveland was given some kind of injection the night before the
operation to help him sleep better—but W. W. Keen later asserted that
the president "passed a good night, sleeping well without any sleeping
medicine." And Edwards mentions nothing of the second, less serious
operation on Cleveland, which Hasbrouck had not participated in and
presumably had no knowledge of.

Nonetheless, the report was, by any measure, an incredibly accurate
account of what was supposed to be a secret medical procedure. And
unlike the cancer rumors that had circulated shortly after the operation,
Edwards's report was clearly substantiated by an eyewitness. Even some
of the drama's principal figures were impressed with Edwards's effort—
though they could never admit that openly. Dan Lamont, who publicly
denounced the report as "infamous," later confided to Edwards that it
was "the greatest news beat." Dr. Keen was equally impressed, calling it
"a great newspaper scoop."

Naturally, Edwards's story was picked up by the wire services and
transmitted to every major newspaper in the country. Many reprinted
it verbatim. By the next day the story was on the front page of papers
from coast to coast, often under hysterical headlines ("He Had a Cancer," shouted the *San Francisco Morning Call*).

In many papers the story appeared alongside reports on the House
vote to repeal the Silver Purchase Act, a juxtaposition that must have
infuriated Cleveland. The stories about his health were overshadowing
one of his greatest political victories.

Dr. Joseph Bryant was none too happy either. He'd always suspected
Ferdinand Hasbrouck was the source of the original cancer rumors. His

suspicions were confirmed by Edwards's report, since it made no mention of the second operation. The leak was Hasbrouck.

Bryant, of course, continued to deny that Cleveland had had a tumor. "The president had some teeth pulled last July, just as I announced after we landed from Mr. Benedict's yacht," Bryant told reporters on the evening that Edwards's story broke. "I will say, however, that President Cleveland, when I saw him last Sunday, was as robust and in as good health as on any day of the ten years in which I have known him."

"I'm afraid that he bent the 10th Commandment rather badly," W. W. Keen later wrote of Bryant, uncharacteristically misidentifying the divine ban on bearing false witness. The other doctors involved in the operation were forced to stretch the limits of truthfulness as well. Bryant's assistant John Erdmann later told Cleveland biographer Allan Nevins that he did more lying during this period than in all the rest of his life put together. Even the pious Keen was forced to fib. Returning from the second operation, he'd bumped into his brother-in-law on the ferry

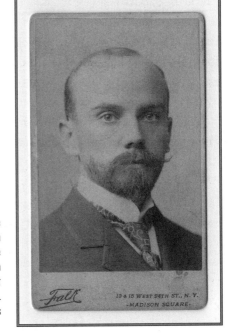

Dr. John Erdmann was just twenty-nine when he assisted in the secret operation on President Cleveland. He would go on to have a long and successful career as a surgeon in New York City, and he would be the last surviving witness to the operation. NYU SCHOOL OF MEDICINE, EHRMAN MEDICAL LIBRARY, ARCHIVES

from Fall River to New York. Asked what he was doing, Keen replied disingenuously that he'd simply had a "consultation" near Newport.

When the story broke, Cleveland was still at Gray Gables, ostensibly recovering from the "strain" he had been under since reassuming the presidency. To discredit the Edwards report, Cleveland once again recruited his friends to lie for him. L. Clarke Davis, the editor of the *Philadelphia Public Ledger*, was enlisted to write an open letter to the papers. "The president's ill health has a real basis of a toothache," Davis wrote. "If it has any other, Mr. Cleveland's closest friends do not know. . . . The president is in excellent health." Davis had a summer home near Gray Gables, and the two men often fished together on Buzzards Bay. Surely he knew the president had suffered from something much more serious than a toothache.

"All the sensational reports about the serious illness of the president are sheer nonsense," Don Dickinson, postmaster general in Cleveland's first administration, told reporters after visiting Gray Gables. "Why, he never looked or felt better in his life."

Elias Benedict told a reporter for Pulitzer's *World* that reports that the president had had cancer were "all rot." The president had merely had a tooth extracted, he said, and "a piece of the jaw bone came away." Asked about reports that the procedure had incapacitated the president for more than a day, Benedict huffed, "All bosh!" "We played [cribbage] every day," Benedict insisted, "and the president never missed a meal."

The *World* even managed to track down Charles Peterson, the *Oneida* steward who had acted as an orderly during the operation. Presumably Peterson was more susceptible than Cleveland's doctors and friends to financial inducements from the yellow papers—a common tactic. But even the steward clung tenaciously to the fiction that nothing dramatic had happened on the yacht during the first week of July. "The president was on deck every day," said Peterson. "I saw him there myself."*

Only Ferdinand Hasbrouck broke the silence. The dentist was the only person with intimate knowledge of the operation to publicly speak

---

* W. W. Keen later noted that the steward received "scant credit" for keeping the secret.

about it at the time. Why did he break his promise? Perhaps, when first confronted by Edwards, he honestly believed—as the newspaperman had led him to believe—that the beans had already been spilled by one of the other doctors involved. Perhaps he simply enjoyed the attention. Maybe he just didn't want to lie anymore. In any event, as far as the rest of the insiders were concerned, he'd betrayed them. "He certainly talked a great deal more than he should have," wrote Keen with typical restraint.

Hasbrouck has his defenders, however. Douglas Barber, a dental historian, believes that, from the beginning, Hasbrouck was the "fall guy" in this game of political intrigue. "If the patient died," Barber writes, "they would proclaim that he had killed the president with his black gas. If the president survived as a vocal cripple, they could blame it on bad dentistry. The phrase 'a bad case of dentistry' had already been used to supplement the official line about the president's rheumatism." Barber blames a bias against dentists for their "advanced ideas about anesthesia" at the time and believes "Hasbrouck surely does not deserve to be called the villain."

On August 30, the day after the Edwards report was published in the *Press*, Cleveland once again left Gray Gables to return to Washington. At his side was Frances, now well into her ninth month of pregnancy, who made the long trip in the searing heat without complaint. Perhaps it would be unfair to suggest that Cleveland exploited his wife's condition, but her conspicuous presence did serve as a convenient counterbalance to questions about his health. In fact, the whole trip was carefully orchestrated to demonstrate Cleveland's vigor. In New York, he made a point of walking from the ferry terminal to the train station, instead of riding in a carriage, as was his custom.

"The president seems a trifle thinner than he was a year ago," the *New York Times* reported the next day, "but on his face is a ruddy glow. His step last evening was elastic, his carriage erect and his actions bespoke a person enjoying perfect health. . . . His face and hands were well browned by his outdoor exercise at Buzzards Bay."

"A bright light was falling upon Mr. Cleveland's face for more than ten minutes," the *World* noted, "and every feature was clear and distinct.

There was no sign of any operation. There was no swelling, no depression. When he spoke he uttered his words clearly and distinctly, unlike a man part of whose jawbone had been removed. His eyes were bright and clear and he seemed cheerful and contented."

Two days later, on September 1, Dr. Bryant examined the president in Washington and pronounced him "all healed." Indeed his progress was extraordinary. The wound in his mouth was completely mended, so Grover could wear his oral prosthesis comfortably for long periods of time. But in other ways, the president was not "all healed," and side effects from the operation would plague him for the rest of his life.

Back in Washington, there were more conspicuous displays of vitality as the president embarked on his most ambitious public schedule since the operation. On the night of September 2, he went to the New National Theater to see a comedy called *The Other Man.*

"The president looked very well indeed," the *New York Times* reported, "and he joined heartily in the laughter." The *Chicago Daily Tribune* noted that, after the play, Cleveland and his companions walked back to the White House "briskly."

Meanwhile, the White House was being inundated with unsolicited "cures" for the president. Letters poured in, prescribing everything from eating "plain food" to going to Colorado for a week or two to "limber up," although Colorado, which was rabidly pro-silver, was probably the last place on Earth that Grover wanted to go.

A concerned citizen from Chicago sent this advice:

> I do not know what truth there may be in the stories of the cancerous nature of the president's late difficulty and do not seek any *ex cathedra* knowledge, but I know of a remedy, thoroughly investigated by me, used under my personal observation with great success, and used by my wife to her own recovery from a most virulent and protracted attack. The remedy consists simply of a tonic . . . it is made chiefly of old-fashioned herbs, is pleasant to take, harmless in every way, and is little known because the compounder, a physician of good education, does not realize the

value, or have the capital to push the remedy. I stumbled on it by accident myself.

The remedy is invented and put up by Dr. S. Brumbaugh of Dayton, Ohio. If the president has any trouble of a cancerous nature, I am sure this man's remedy will stop all pain and effect a radical cure. The doctor is rather a rattle-headed fellow, but he *has found a cancer cure* [emphasis in original]. It is a case where "these things are withheld from the wise and revealed unto babes."

I should consider it a great public calamity at this time if anything should take President Cleveland from the helm.

Cleveland faced his biggest test on September 6, when he hosted a White House reception for hundreds of doctors attending the Pan-American Medical Congress in Washington. He passed with flying colors. The president mingled among the doctors, none of whom detected any sign of surgery having been performed on him. He even gave a short speech, praising "those who devote themselves to saving human life and to the alleviation of human suffering." His voice was described as clear and articulate. Some said the president hadn't sounded so good since his inauguration. He seemed to be the picture of health.

9

LIAR

WHEN E. J. EDWARDS left the *New York Sun* for the *Philadelphia Press* in 1889, he traded one newspaper war for another. The competition for readers was no less intense in Philadelphia than it was in New York, and no two papers in the City of Brotherly Love competed more fiercely than the *Press* and the *Times*.

Press publisher Charles Emory Smith was Philly's version of Charles Dana, an erudite New Englander infatuated with the English language. "The readers of the *Press* are familiar with his style," a contemporary wrote, "a clear, strong variety of English which admits of no beating around the bush." Born in 1842, Smith was just sixteen when he began his newspaper career writing editorials for the *Albany Evening Transcript*. In 1861 he graduated from Union College in Schenectady and became a recruiting officer for the Union Army. After the war he worked at newspapers in Albany before purchasing an interest in the *Press* in 1880.

Smith's bitter antagonist was Alexander K. McClure, the quixotic publisher of the *Times* and Philadelphia's answer to Joseph Pulitzer. Born on a farm in Perry County, Pennsylvania, in 1828, McClure had little formal schooling and went to work at fourteen as a tanner's apprentice. In his teens he also began freelancing for the *Perry Freemason*, the local newspaper, and at nineteen he was appointed the paper's editor. Three years later McClure headed a group of investors who bought a newspaper in Chambersburg, Pennsylvania, called the *Franklin Repository*.

Originally a Whig, McClure was an early convert to the Republican Party. In 1853, when he was just twenty-five, McClure was the party's candidate for Pennsylvania auditor general, the youngest nominee for a statewide office in Pennsylvania at that time. He lost, but four years later he was elected to the state legislature, becoming one of the first Republicans seated in that body.

At the Republican National Convention in 1860, McClure helped swing the Pennsylvania delegation to Lincoln, and as the party's state chairman in Pennsylvania, he was instrumental in helping Lincoln carry that pivotal state. For this, Lincoln was deeply grateful, and it was said that McClure had a standing invitation to the White House when Lincoln was president.

The *Franklin Repository* was a Republican newspaper, naturally, and during the Civil War it was one of the most prominent antislavery papers in Pennsylvania. McClure was merciless in his condemnation of the rebels, who exacted their revenge in 1864 when Confederate troops burned Chambersburg to the ground, specifically targeting McClure's home.

After the war McClure moved to Philadelphia, and in 1875 he founded the *Times* with a friend named Frank McLaughlin. Their initial investment was $50,000. Within ten years the paper was worth a million. McClure mimicked Pulitzer in many ways. The *Times* was heavy on sensationalism and illustrations, and the paper organized Pulitzer-like publicity stunts, such as raising $7,000 from readers to underwrite an "old time" Fourth of July celebration in 1887. But McClure was not merely an imitator. The *Times* was also one of the first newspapers to experiment with banner headlines, and the paper crusaded relentlessly against corruption in city government. McClure was sued for libel twenty times by the targets of his investigations. Not one of those cases was successful. McClure introduced Philadelphia to an aggressive brand of journalism that left his competitors—particularly the staid *Press*—scrambling to catch up.

In the 1870s, McClure drifted away from the Republican Party. Appalled by the remorseless corruption of the Grant administration, he helped organize the Liberal Republicans, a breakaway faction that nominated *New York Tribune* editor Horace Greeley to run for president in 1872. (Greeley, of course, was trounced, and he died just twenty-four days after the election.) In 1880, McClure abandoned the Republicans altogether and supported Democrat Winfield Scott Hancock for president. Four years later, he endorsed Grover Cleveland.

Just as he had helped Lincoln get elected in 1860, Alexander McClure helped Cleveland get elected in 1884. It was in McClure's hotel room at the Democratic convention that Pennsylvania's party bosses agreed to support Cleveland's nomination—in exchange for control of patronage in the state.

A month after the election, McClure went to Albany to meet Cleveland for the first time. He found him to be a "quiet, unassuming, straightforward, sternly honest and entirely frank man," as well as a "delightful conversationalist." McClure recommended himself to Cleveland chiefly by asking no favors. "I had no favorites to press upon him for any position," McClure wrote, "and that probably brought me into closer personal connection with him during his later career than could have been obtained had I annoyed him with the claims of placemen." The two men forged what McClure called "an intimate acquaintance," and McClure frequently visited Cleveland when he was president. "I have many times gone to the White House by his appointment after ten o'clock at night," McClure wrote, "and often passed the midnight hour with him."

McClure was one of the few newspapermen admitted to Cleveland's inner circle, and he supported the president unconditionally. The *Times*, of course, played the same tune as its publisher, and even as the economy imploded in 1893, the paper steadfastly backed Cleveland. The

Times was in denial about the panic, continually insisting things were getting better, or at least weren't as bad as they seemed. Among the paper's headlines that summer: "Hard Times Are Over." "Things Have Been Exaggerated." "Outlook Better Than Last Year." "The Depression Is Over." It was the journalism of wishful thinking.

When E. J. Edwards published his explosive account of the secret operation performed on Cleveland, McClure leaped to his friend's defense. McClure, who lived on a farm outside Philadelphia, liked to call himself a farmer, though his friends joked that his only crops were "sarcasm, irony, and invective." All three would be harvested plentifully by McClure to attack his archrival the *Press*, as well as E. J. Edwards personally.

It was not an era of good manners in journalism. Much like today's cable news channels, newspapers competed ruthlessly for their audiences in a market that was hopelessly oversaturated. In the spring of 1870 there emerged what the newspaper historian Frank Luther Mott describes as an "epidemic of vituperation" among the New York dailies. "We observe that most of the newspapers in this city and Brooklyn have allowed themselves during the past week to attack each other in a highly personal manner," read an editorial in the *Tribune*. "Why cannot Editors learn that the public wants of them nothing but the publication of news and temperate, dignified, gentlemanly explanation and criticism of current events?" Not that the *Tribune* was above the fray. Less than two weeks earlier the paper had said of the *New York Times*, "[It] lies deliberately, willfully, wickedly, and with naked intent to defame and malign."

Twenty-three years later, E. J. Edwards's report triggered a similar epidemic in Philadelphia.

On August 30, 1893, the day after Edwards's story appeared in the *Press*, the *Times* began a systematic campaign to discredit it—and E. J. Edwards. Page one carried a report from Washington quoting Henry Thurber, one of the president's secretaries. "I hear from Mr. Cleveland nearly every day," Thurber said, "and in all of his letters he speaks of his improving health and strength. . . . Bills and other matters that require his signature are received by me almost daily, and the president's name is signed in a hand that shows health and vigor." Hardly irrefutable evidence of good health, but enough for the *Times* correspondent to pronounce the story of his "alleged" illness "discredited." The *Times'* lead editorial that day was entitled, "The Panic-Monger's Degradation." Almost certainly penned by McClure himself, the editorial scathingly, sarcastically attacks Edwards and his report:

> In conscienceless sensationalism we recall nothing more infamous than a long dispatch printed yesterday by the *Press* under the date of New York with the displayed heading, "The President a Very Sick Man." It professes to reveal, with great regret and under a stern sense of duty, some awful facts about the president that his friends have concealed. . . . [Edwards] builds up three columns of pretentious and portentous verbiage and sneaking insinuation. He hopes that it is not cancer. True, there is no reason to suppose that it is, but then General Grant died of cancer. And Mr. Cleveland is so noble, so heroic, so beloved; it would be a calamity for the country to lose him; and all this in a tone of fulsome insincerity that is all the viler because so plausible. . . .
>
> But we can have no quarrel with a person of this sort. It is not the writing of his sensations that we object to, but the printing of them, and for that the responsibility belongs to the paper that for weeks and months has been laboring by every device of exaggeration, misrepresentation, or suppression, by distorting news or by making it, to excite a panic among its readers. . . . The best that can be said of this latest sensation is that it seems to mark the lowest depth to which it is possible even for the *Press* to sink.

McClure did not let up. The front page of the next day's *Times* carried a rare banner headline: "The President Is All Right, The Country Is All Right, Business Will Be All Right." Underneath it—and a subhead reading "The Calamity-Howler's Lies"—the *Times* published a story that begins, "The only element of truth in the latest story of

President Cleveland's illness which has been printed in Philadelphia is that he suffered from toothache and that the teeth which pained him were removed on board E. C. Benedict's yacht."

"A Mr. Edwards, of the Philadelphia *Press*," the story continues, "discovered that the president had been in a dentist's chair and he surrounded his report of that event with all the cruel and cold-blooded details, true and false, which his imagination could call up."

The story repeats the administration's lie that the president had merely had some dental work performed upon him on the yacht:

> During the evening of the first day out Dr. Hasbrouck removed two teeth from Mr. Cleveland's jaw. Dr. Keen assisted him in one of the commonest, simplest operations known to dentistry when he cut away a part of the antrum of the jaw which had been diseased along with the teeth. There was no question of cancer or of sarcoma, and the cutting away of the diseased tissue was an operation which dentists find necessary in nine out of every ten cases of this kind which come before them. The comparison between Mr. Cleveland's toothache and the serious malady from which General Grant suffered and which caused his death was only another evidence of the exquisite heartlessness of the newspaper correspondent. . . .
>
> If anything further is needed to refute this and future stories of Mr. Cleveland's health it is an exact understanding of their source. . . . When Mr. Cleveland made his trip on the *Oneida* to Buzzards Bay, Mr. Edwards recorded the journey pleasantly, and his account of it written at the time is today the best evidence of the deliberate falsity of his second report.

A *Times* editorial entitled "A Disgrace to Journalism" once again excoriates Edwards. The correspondent "twists and obscures" the facts to "bolster up the original lie." "This sort of misreporting is the very depth of despicable journalism." McClure was unrelenting. The next day, September 1, the *Times* published a cartoon on the front page that

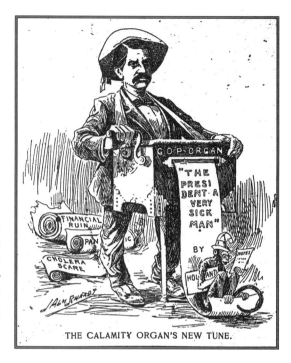

This editorial cartoon appeared on the front page of the *Philadelphia Times* on September 1, 1893. It was part of *Times* publisher Alexander McClure's campaign to discredit E. J. Edwards and his story about the secret operation on the president.

FREE LIBRARY OF PHILADELPHIA

THE CALAMITY ORGAN'S NEW TUNE.

depicts the GOP as an organ grinder and Edwards as the organ grinder's monkey. Under the headline "The Calamity Liar," it also published an interview Ferdinand Hasbrouck gave the *New York Tribune*, emphasizing minor inconsistencies that supposedly proved Edwards had "faked" his original interview with the dentist. The paper also reprinted L. Clarke Davis's "toothache" letter claiming the president was "in excellent health." In the following days the *Times* labeled Edwards a "calamity howler" and a "famous falsifier" and accused him of committing "crimes against public tranquility."

Other papers also questioned the veracity of Edwards's report. The *Philadelphia Inquirer* dismissed it as "not a new story." But none attacked with the venom of the *Times*. As Edwards himself wrote many years later, "I was very grossly abused, especially by the Phila. *Times*."

Times publisher Alexander McClure seems to have taken this particular battle quite personally. At the very least he was unsportsmanlike. Partly this was due to his friendship with Cleveland, but it was also because he simply loathed the *Press* and its editor, Charles Emory Smith. The *Press* epitomized much that McClure despised about the newspaper business. It was stuffy and pompous, and its editor, in McClure's opinion, was an unctuous jerk with an unwarranted overabundance of self-esteem.

Likewise, McClure could not abide the college-educated reporters then in their ascendency in the newspaper business—reporters like E. J. Edwards, a Yale grad twice over. After all, McClure himself had left school by the time he was fourteen. As far as he was concerned, college was a waste of time for journalists. In an 1877 editorial he advised young men considering a career in newspapers that "journalism is the most exacting of all professions, and the sooner young men dismiss the idea that a college diploma qualifies them to take an editorial or reporter's chair the sooner they will protect themselves against every disappointment." McClure resented the growing influence of college men in the newspaper business, and he took it out on E. J. Edwards.

The *Times'* mistreatment of Edwards must have appalled Dr. William Williams Keen, the good Baptist. Undoubtedly the vitriol offended his sense of Christian charity, but he felt powerless to intervene. Torn between his vow of secrecy and a desire to vindicate Edwards, Keen chose to honor the former at the cost of the reporter's reputation. Keen would never quite forgive himself for failing to speak out in the journalist's defense.

At first Edwards's paper dismissed the *Times* attacks as unworthy of a response. "As for the Philadelphia *Times*," a *Press* editorial from August 31 says, "we have only to say that it has ceased to be a newspaper and become chiefly a stockjobbing concern, and its treatment of this subject is beneath contempt." (The term "stockjobber" referred to an unscrupulous stockbroker.) But the following day, the *Press* promised to start fighting back. "The *Times* has chosen, spitefully, pettishly, indecently, with the single interest of a stockjobber and the venom of a rattlesnake, to strike at the *Press*. We never open that kind of a fight, but we never shrink from it." The editorial called the *Times* "stupid," "malignant," and "asinine."

The next day the *Times* responded with a warning. "The *Press* should keep its temper," the paper said. "Impetuous bombast won't hide or excuse the terrible blunder that journal has committed in its calamity falsehood about the fatal illness of the President."

The *Press* fired back:

> We beg the pardon of our readers for a method of treatment in this case which is not according to our usual standard and taste. But there is a kind of animal with which it is difficult to hold honorable controversy. There are only two ways of dealing with it. The first is to leave its own field to itself, and keep out of reach of the filth. The other is to accept the risk of unpleasant contact and do a little straight, downright clubbing for the common weal. There are times when the latter alternative, however unwelcome, is a real public service. . . .
>
> The opinion or attitude of the *Times* as to the *Press* publication concerning the President was not in itself of the slightest consequence. . . . But however impotent the rage, however pitiful the jealousy and however inconsequential the harmfulness of the *Times*, the *Press* is not in the habit of letting such vicious attacks, come from what source they may, go unrebuked. . . .
>
> There was no reasonable warrant or justification for any criticism upon the *Press* in connection with Holland's publication. . . . There is not a real metropolitan newspaper of enterprise in New York or Boston or Chicago that would not gladly have paid at least $1000 for its exclusive possession and publication, and every journalist knows it. Through the confidence which Holland has carefully built up by his long and honorable work, it happened to fall into the possession of the metropolitan newspaper of Philadelphia, and its careful publication in the most conservative manner was not only an illustration of the best journalism, but it was a distinct

public service because it cleared away a cloud of rumors and mysteries and perplexities, and presented the truth which it is always best to meet and to face. . . .

Enough said. Au revoir.

Two days later, on Tuesday, September 5, the *Times* published another editorial cartoon on page one. This one depicts McClure as a doctor amputating Edwards's right foot and left arm, which are wrapped in bandages marked "Presidential Cancer" and "Panic."

The caption: "Au Revoir!"

The battle between the *Press* and the *Times* became a story in its own right, with other papers taking sides. "The Boss Flunker is the Philadelphia *Times*," said the *Harrisburg Telegraph*. "McClure made a great play at Charles Emory Smith of the *Press* and blackguarded him like a pickpocket because the *Press* printed the news about Cleveland's illness." Some thought the spat was just plain silly. The *Philadelphia Inquirer* quipped, "The President's health yesterday was just robust enough to give the robust liars on both sides another chance to have him slowly dying and stronger than the strongest man."

More significantly, E. J. Edwards's report and the subsequent dispute between the *Press* and the *Times* touched off an unprecedented national debate over the public's right to know about the health of the president. Until then, no one had paid much heed to a president's wellness (unless he'd been shot). Notoriously sickly chief executives like Andrew Jackson had taken virtually no steps to hide their conditions from the public—Old Hickory had an old bullet wound in his chest that was continually infected and was said to give off a most unappealing odor. But Edwards's report spurred many newspapers to demand President Cleveland come clean about his health. "The people had a right to this information," said New Jersey's *Trenton Gazette*. "President Cleveland belongs to them more than he belongs to himself or his few close friends." Of course, papers sympathetic to the president disagreed. "Grover Cleveland has as much right to privacy as any or every other American citizen," said the *Brooklyn Daily Eagle*. "The President has the right of every other citizen to the protection of his confidences with his physicians, his friends and his family from lugubrious publication."

One thing many papers could agree on was that the president should have been more forthcoming from the start. "If the facts had been frankly and fully stated at the beginning," the *Troy Times* of New York editorialized, "there would have been no occasion for the public uneasiness regarding the President's condition."

Given the conflicting accounts of the president's health, the public was largely inclined to believe that E. J. Edwards had, at the very least, exaggerated the severity of the president's condition. Some even believed he'd made the whole thing up, just as Alexander McClure kept insisting. The Cleveland administration's strategy—constant denials and staged displays of the president's fitness—paid off. Most Americans were probably already inclined to believe the Honest President anyway. Ironically, Cleveland's reputation for integrity actually made it easier for him to pull off one of the great deceptions in American political history.

Even Edwards's peers were inclined to give the president, not the newspaperman, the benefit of the doubt. While acknowledging the "brilliant scope of Mr. Edwards," the trade journal the *Journalist* concluded that "his assertion that the operation was for the removal of a cancerous growth must be set down, at least, as not proven, for while no official denial has been made, the doctors and near friends of Mr. Cleveland say that the operation was simply for the removal of ulcerated teeth and a portion of the jaw bone which had become affected."

Ultimately, E. J. Edwards's reputation was seriously compromised. He had been labeled a "faker," and that label would stick to him for a long time. The criticism was wholly unjustified, of course, but Edwards took it stoically, in a manner befitting a nineteenth-century gentleman. Yet it must have eaten away at him.

Grover Cleveland would also benefit—if that's the right word—from one of the worst natural disasters in American history, which would sweep questions about his health off the front pages.

Around nine o'clock on the night of August 10, 1893, a meteor as big as a barrel streaked across the sky over Savannah, Georgia, and plunged into Wassaw Sound, a coastal bay where the Wilmington River flows into the Atlantic. The impact resonated with a tremendous explosion and sent a geyser of steam rising high into the warm night air. To the Gullah, the African American residents of the Sea Islands off the coasts of Georgia and South Carolina, the meteor was a bad omen. More than one hundred thousand Gullah lived on the islands and the coastal plain, a region known as the Lowcountry. They were former slaves and their descendents, desperately poor and deeply superstitious. The door-frames of their rickety wooden houses were painted bright blue to ward off evil spirits. They believed the meteor, which landed very close to them, portended something sinister. The older Gullah well remembered that August was the month that disastrous storms had swept across their islands in 1856, 1881, 1885, and 1886.

To the white residents of the coastal region, the meteor was nothing more than an unusual if rather frightening meteorological phenome-non. They paid no heed to the superstitions of the Sea Island "darkies."

However, on Tuesday, August 22, just twelve days after the meteor strike, ships sailing into Savannah carried disquieting news: a major storm was brewing off the coast. In fact, as meteorologists would later discover, not one but four hurricanes were swirling simultaneously in the Atlantic that day, an event never before recorded, and one that would not be repeated until 1998. Two of the hurricanes would peter out before causing major damage, but on Wednesday, August 23, one of the storms slammed into New York City with, by one account, "unexampled fury." At least thirty people were killed, mostly sailors whose boats capsized. A thirty-foot storm surge swept across south-ern Brooklyn and Queens, destroying virtually everything in its path. On Coney Island, the elevated railroad was swept away. Hog Island, a mile-long island off Long Island that was a playground for the rich and famous, was completely obliterated. It literally vanished overnight. The 1893 New York hurricane remains one of the most destructive storms in U.S. history.

Yet it was nothing compared to the storm that would hit the Sea Islands just four days later.

Even before those ships had sailed into Savannah with news of the storm, Lewis N. Jesunofsky, a Weather Bureau forecaster in the city, suspected something serious was afoot in the Atlantic. The barometric pressure was falling precipitously, and wind speeds were rising ominously. Jesunofsky knew he had to warn residents of the impending storm, but his options were limited. Red and black hurricane flags were hoisted above government buildings. Bulletins were posted on telegraph poles. Perhaps he mailed a few postcards to the outlying islands. Local newspapers were little help. On Saturday, August 26, the *Savannah Morning News* carried a small item headlined, "Another Storm Coming." It appeared on the bottom of page eight. By the time most Sea Islanders realized how destructive the storm would be, it was far too late.

It made landfall on the afternoon of Sunday, August 27. The eye passed over Savannah around 10:00 P.M. More than ten inches of rain fell that night, with winds reaching 120 miles per hour. The storm surge was estimated to be anywhere from sixteen to thirty feet. Under the modern classification system, the storm was a Category 3 hurricane. In Beaufort, South Carolina, about twenty miles north of Savannah, the tide was eight feet higher than normal, with waves of twenty feet. The storm raged for fourteen hours. "Sunday night was a night of sheer terror," write Bill and Fran Marscher in *The Great Sea Island Storm of 1893*. "Those who lived through it never forgot it."

When dawn broke on Monday, August 28, the scene was one of appalling devastation. The low-lying Sea Islands were swamped. As many as two thousand people, mostly Gullah, were dead. Hundreds had been washed out to sea, never to be seen again. The Sea Island hurricane still stands as the third or fourth deadliest in U.S. history. The Gullah's houses were smashed to splinters. Some thirty thousand people were rendered homeless. The corn and potato crops, the Gullah's main source of sustenance, were ruined. They had no drinking water, for their wells had been contaminated with seawater. These were the poorest people in one of the poorest states in a nation crippled by depression—and now what little they had had was gone. One eyewitness said, "Death and destruction seemed triumphant all around." In Gullah folklore the storm would be remembered as "de big blow."

This already isolated region was now completely cut off from the rest of the world. It took four days for a message from the Sea Islands to reach South Carolina governor Ben Tillman. The telegram begged for "speedy relief." Tillman's reply was hardly encouraging. He appealed for donations of food and clothing but warned the Gullah that he did not want any "abuse of charity." "We want to guard against those people who, seeing that aid is coming, might do nothing."

Pitchfork Ben, as he liked to call himself in a transparent homage to farmers, was a notorious racist. In 1900 he would brag about how effectively South Carolina had managed to disenfranchise African Americans: "We stuffed ballot boxes. We shot them. We are not ashamed of it." He was not inclined to go out of his way to help the Gullah. "The people have the fish of the sea there to prevent them from starving," he said. Of course, the people had neither boats nor nets to fish with. They had all been destroyed in the storm.

Given Grover Cleveland's aversion to "paternalism," it's not surprising that the federal government was no more responsive. When Senator Matthew Butler of South Carolina appealed to Secretary of War Dan Lamont for assistance, Lamont said it would be unconstitutional for the government to provide direct aid, though he did offer to lend some spare tents to the homeless. It was a principled position, though not a very popular one, and it did little to endear Grover Cleveland to a public grown weary of the panic.

Three weeks after the storm hit, Clara Barton inspected the region at the request of Governor Tillman and Senator Butler. Barton had founded the American Red Cross as a disaster relief organization twelve years earlier. She had seen her share of tragedies, but nothing prepared her for what she encountered on the Sea Islands. Bloated corpses were still lying in muddy fields. There were no shovels to bury the bodies, and even if there had been, the people were too weak to dig. More numerous were the carcasses of cows and horses killed under collapsed barns or drowned in pastures. Malaria was already rampant. Simply cleaning up would be an enormous undertaking; rebuilding, even more so. But the most pressing needs were the most basic: food, clothing, shelter.

Although she was seventy-two, Barton organized the relief effort with the energy of a woman half her age. She commandeered two large warehouses in Beaufort for a command post. She determined that "a fixed system of relief must be adopted, a rigid economy enforced," and "every person who could do so must be made to work for his food and receive food and raiment only in return for labor." She appealed to Northern newspapers for help, and soon trains and boats laden with donated goods were steaming into Beaufort. For the papers, the hurricane was a bonanza, providing them with sensational stories of death and survival, as well as a crusade. Hurricane relief became a cause célèbre. Newspapers practically tripped over each other in publishing appeals for donation. Not to be outdone, Pulitzer's *World* even commissioned a train to deliver donated supplies, which were sorted at the warehouses and then delivered by small boats to the islanders.

The Red Cross would have to feed as many as seventy-five thousand people for eight months, until the spring crops could be harvested. "The charge was immense," Barton wrote. "Not alone the welfare, the lives of these thousands of human beings would be in our hands." The rations were necessarily meager: eight quarts of hominy grits and one pound of pork per week for a family of seven. But it was enough to survive.

The Red Cross also struggled to restore the landscape. To earn their rations, able-bodied men were put to work digging ditches to drain the islands, planting crops, and, with donated lumber and tools, building new houses, first for widows and the infirm.

The winter passed. It was hard, but there was no famine. In the spring, the corn and potatoes returned. The Red Cross distributed its last rations in May 1894. In September, the organization departed. Barton believed it was just as important to know when to end relief efforts as when to begin them.

The hurricane had pummeled the Sea Islands just two days before E. J. Edwards published his beat on August 29. As the enormity of the tragedy became apparent, stories from the Sea Islands pushed reports about the secret operation on the president out of the papers. The timing of the tragedy was perfect for purposes of the cover-up.

Then something happened that would put questions about Grover's health to rest for good.

———•••———

On the morning of Saturday, September 9, a "general air of expectancy" permeated the White House. The doorkeepers and valets walked on tiptoes across the marble floors. Grover was behind his massive *Resolute* desk as usual, but he was clearly preoccupied. Just down the hall, in the master bedroom, Frances was in labor. Dr. Bryant was with her, and occasionally he would scribble a message on a small slip of paper and have it delivered to the president. Between these updates, Grover, as anxious as any expectant father, pretended to work. At eleven o'clock he sent a note to Dan Lamont at the War Department. The Marine Band was scheduled to perform a public concert on the White House lawn that afternoon. Grover asked Lamont to cancel it.

Childbirth was a dangerous endeavor in 1893. It killed one out of every one hundred women giving birth. (Today the rate in developed nations is one out of every ten thousand women.) Obstetrics was just emerging as a medical specialty. Physicians had begun replacing midwives, but only among the upper classes. Obstetrical wards had been established in some hospitals in the 1880s, though only the urban poor, whose homes were generally small and unhygienic, gave birth in hospitals. Women of means would not begin having children in hospitals in large numbers until well into the twentieth century.

While we can never know for certain the details of what happened in the master bedroom that morning, it's safe to assume that certain Gilded Age conventions were adhered to. Even in the intimacy of childbirth, modesty ruled the relationship between doctor and patient. It's likely Frances gave birth lying on her side with her knees pulled up to her chest. This is known as the Sims' position, named for J. Marion Sims, a nineteenth-century physician who pioneered advances in gynecology, though this progress came at the expense of the enslaved women on whom he experimented. In the Sims' position, the mother can avoid eye contact with the doctor, thereby preserving her dignity, the reasoning went. Dr. Bryant, meanwhile, would be expected to avert his eyes from the main event. Doctors were encouraged to deliver babies "by touch," so as to avoid offending women by looking at their genitalia.

By this cumbersome process, a healthy baby girl was delivered at noon. A few minutes later, Grover was summoned to the bedroom. Bryant informed him that Mrs. Cleveland had given birth to a "remarkably healthy and vigorous" girl. The mother, he said, was doing "wonderfully well." The two men then shook hands warmly. Grover asked the doctor to keep the news to himself for the time being. Then he visited his wife and their newborn for about fifteen minutes before returning to his desk.

At two o'clock that afternoon, Grover finally broadcast the news. He informed his cabinet, and one of his secretaries told an Associated Press correspondent, "You can tell the world that we have a little girl baby here." Soon telegrams and letters of congratulations were pouring in. The Clevelands would receive more than seventeen thousand in all. In a rare display of leniency, Grover gave the White House staff the rest of the day off.

The second Cleveland daughter was the first and thus far only child of a president to be born in the White House itself, though she was not the first baby born there. Nine other children had already entered the world within the historic walls of the presidential mansion. The first was Thomas Jefferson's grandson, James Madison Randolph, in 1806. John Quincy Adams and Ulysses Grant each welcomed a grandchild there. John Tyler greeted two. And Andrew Jackson's niece Emily Donelson gave birth to four children in the White House. Since the birth of the Cleveland daughter, however, only one other baby has been born in the White House: Woodrow Wilson's grandson, Francis B. Sayre Jr., in 1915. Sayre became a prominent minister, serving twenty-seven years as dean of the National Cathedral in Washington. He died in 2008.

Since the Clevelands already had a daughter, many Americans had hoped their second child would be a boy. "When the news that the . . . child was a girl spread through the city," one paper reported, "there were many expressions of disappointment." The proud parents, however, couldn't have been happier. "She is a sweet baby," Frances wrote to a friend, "looking much as Ruth did at her age, with dark eyes and hair. All here are pleased that she is a girl, however disappointed the nation may be."

Six days later, the Clevelands announced the baby's name: Esther. The papers said the name carried no special significance "other than the partiality of the parents for Scriptural denominatives." (In the Old Testament, Esther is a queen, the wife of King Ahasuerus.) It was also noted that the name means "star." Even in 1893 the name was considered old-fashioned, and, unlike with her older sister, Esther's birth did not inspire a wave of namesakes. Between 1892 and 1894, the name only rose from sixty-seventh to thirty-sixth on the list of most popular names for baby girls. Still, it was a fine name. "The president's babies are happily named," opined the *Richmond Dispatch*. "Ruth and Esther go well together, and they are short, sensible, and nonpartisan names."

The birth of Esther seemed to prove that Cleveland was healthy—even virile—and apparently settled the matter once and for all: the president was not a sick man.

On September 11, two days after the birth, Grover wrote his friend Thomas Bayard, who was the American ambassador to Britain. In this unusually personal letter, Grover discussed his health and E. J. Edwards's report in the *Philadelphia Press*. These are his only words on the matter known to have survived.

> The report you saw regarding my health resulted from a most astounding breach of professional duty on the part of a medical man [Ferdinand Hasbrouck]. I tell you this in strict confidence, for the policy here has been to deny and discredit his story. I believe the American public and newspapers are not speculating further on the subject.

The truth is, officeseeking and officeseekers came very near putting a period to my public career. Whatever else developed found its opportunity in the weakened walls of a constitution that had long withstood fierce attacks. I turned the corner to the stage of enforced care-taking almost in a day. And this must be hereafter the condition on which will depend my health and life. Another phase of the situation cannot be spoken of with certainty, but I believe the chances in my favor are at least even.

I have learned how weak the strongest man is under God's decrees and I see in a new light the necessity of doing my allotted work in the full apprehension of the coming night.

You must understand that I am regarded here as a perfectly well man and the story of an important surgical operation is thoroughly discredited. I think I never looked better and I am much stronger than I have lately been. You have now more of the story than anyone else outside of the medical circle.

PART III

VINDICATION

10

AFTERMATH

HOSEA PERKINS was a millionaire who lived in a mansion in Washington Heights, a neighborhood on the north end of Manhattan. He'd made his fortune in the carpet business. After he retired, he indulged his passion for learning by earning degrees from Bowdoin College and Dartmouth. He started a second career as an orator and was much in demand as an after-dinner speaker. He was also famous for his Independence Day speeches. His neighbors called him the Sage of Washington Heights.

Hosea was an early riser, and on the morning of Tuesday, September 12, 1893, he was out of bed by six o'clock as usual. He opened the bedroom blinds, and in the dawning light he saw a man sleeping on his front lawn. Perturbed, he donned a robe and slippers and went outside to rouse the vagrant. It probably wasn't the first time a wayward drunk had made himself comfortable on Hosea Perkins's luxuriant lawn.

Stepping out his front door, Hosea called out to the prostrate stranger but got no answer. As he moved closer to him, Hosea was surprised to see the man was dressed in a fine suit. Beside him was a lovely silver-tipped cane. The cane looked familiar to Hosea.

A bolt of panic shot through the old man.

While Grover Cleveland endeavored to project an air of vigor, other Americans were struggling with the urge to kill themselves. Reliable statistics are hard to come by, but anecdotal evidence suggests the suicide rate increased dramatically during the Panic of 1893. In May, the *New York Tribune* published an editorial entitled, "Epidemics of Suicide." "During the last fortnight there has been an unusually heavy record of mortality from this cause in New York and Brooklyn," the paper said. Noting that five cases had been reported just the day before, the *Tribune* speculated, "There must be something in the social environment and in the spirit of the times that serves to deepen the overshadowing gloom . . . and to inspire the suicidal impulse."

"Suicides seem to be constantly on the increase," the *St. Paul Daily Globe* noted in September. "The existing financial crisis has contributed largely to this increase."

Hosea Perkins's eldest son, Edwin, enjoyed life. Still a bachelor at forty-two, Edwin lived in Harlem, where he was a "conspicuous figure" and "kept very lively company." He was said to possess "an impulsive, warm-hearted temperament . . . and fine literary abilities." Edwin was a stockbroker, and he was well known on Wall Street. For several years he'd held a seat on the New York Stock Exchange, but in 1889 he traded it for one on the Consolidated Exchange. His timing couldn't have been worse. Known as the Little Board, the Consolidated Exchange specialized in mining and oil stocks, nearly all of which tanked in the panic. Edwin suffered huge losses, and he was forced to borrow money from his father to fund his extravagant lifestyle.

Still, Edwin seemed to take his misfortune in stride. He visited his father on the evening of September 11. "He showed signs of being somewhat unbalanced," the *New York Tribune* reported, "but his father did not think he was in serious trouble." Later that night Edwin returned to his apartment in Harlem. He put on his best black suit and a pair of fancy dress gloves. He picked up his favorite cane, the one with the silver tip. And he slipped a small, .32-caliber pistol into his pocket.

He went back to his father's house. Standing on the lawn, he raised the gun to his right temple and pulled the trigger. He left no note.

Moments after Hosea discovered his son dead on the lawn, the paperboy arrived with the morning paper. Hosea was kneeling beside the body, holding Edwin's head on his knees. The boy helped Hosea carry the body inside the house. About thirty minutes later a policeman making his rounds was stopped by one of Hosea's servants and informed of the shooting. The investigation was perfunctory. The coroner ruled the death a suicide, and at four o'clock that afternoon, Hosea was issued a permit to bury his son.

Hosea had no doubt that his son had killed himself over his financial problems. He said his son "had been affected by financial losses caused by the stringency in the money market." A private funeral was held on September 14. Edwin was buried in Woodlawn Cemetery.

Certainly, Edwin Perkins was not the only businessman driven to suicide in 1893. On October 25, Nathan Strauss, the New York representative of Levi Strauss, shot himself in the head in his office. Strauss, who was Levi's nephew, had reportedly suffered heavy losses in railroad stocks. No less tragic were the more humble suicides. John Baptist Dunne, a thirty-year-old bachelor despondent over losing his job as a clerk at American Express and unable to provide for his widowed mother, shot himself inside a Catholic church in New York after attending Mass on December 1.

The epidemic did not escape the notice of President Cleveland, who not only read of suicides in the papers but was also touched by the phenomenon, at least indirectly.

In the early afternoon of July 8, 1893, a fifty-year-old politician named Charles Perry walked into a Buffalo cemetery. Perry was from Mt. Morris, a western New York town about sixty miles east of Buffalo, so Grover must have known him fairly well. Perry was experiencing "financial difficulties," and he'd told his family he was headed to Buffalo on business. Standing on the bank of a picturesque lake in the cemetery, Perry put the muzzle of a revolver in his mouth and pulled the trigger. He fell into the lake but was quickly pulled out of the water by several alert groundskeepers. Amazingly, Perry survived. The bullet had passed through his upper jaw and exited his left ear, missing his brain completely. His poor marksmanship saved his life.

Of course, desperation did not always lead to attempts at self-destruction. More often it led to agitation and confrontation. Employers responded to the panic by laying off workers in droves and slashing the wages of those who remained. In the railroad, mining, and textile industries, wages fell by as much as 50 percent, while the workday was routinely lengthened from eight hours to ten. Workers had little recourse. Organized labor was anything but organized in 1893. A strike at a steel mill in Homestead, Pennsylvania, the previous year had been brutally crushed, leaving the movement demoralized. A hodgepodge of specialized unions competed with each other for pieces of a rapidly shrinking pie. For example, there were about eight hundred thousand railroad employees in the United States, of whom some 150,000 belonged to various unions: switchmen, engineers, firemen, conductors, station men, shop workers. Among these factions there was virtually no cooperation.

Eugene V. Debs thought there was a better way. The son of Alsatian immigrants who settled in Terre Haute, Indiana, Debs was the national secretary-treasurer of the Brotherhood of Locomotive Firemen. He believed all railroad workers should be "under one roof," represented by a single union. So he started one. He quit the firemen's union, and, at a meeting in Chicago on June 20, 1893—right around the time Grover's tumor was first diagnosed—Eugene Debs organized the American Railway Union. Membership was open to anyone who worked for a railroad in any capacity outside management. (Well, anyone who was white. African Americans and other minority groups were excluded by the union's executive board, despite Debs's objections.) Even longshoremen and miners who worked for railroad companies were eligible, as were employees of companies that operated railroads on the side.

Debs made membership affordable. At a time when most unions charged dues of ten to twenty-five dollars a year, the ARU charged members less than two dollars. Despite massive layoffs in the industry, membership took off faster than the New York Central's legendary Engine 999, the fastest steam locomotive in the world at that time, capable of speeds in excess of eighty miles per hour. Within a year, 150,000 workers would belong to the ARU—as many as had belonged to all the other railroad unions combined.

Bald and myopic, Debs did not cut an imposing figure. But he was fearless and beloved by the members of his union. "He was the bravest man I ever knew," labor lawyer Clarence Darrow said of Debs. Darrow was deeply impressed by Debs's personality. "There may have lived some time, somewhere, a kindlier, gentler, more generous man than Eugene Debs, but I have never known him."

Nobody imagined it when the ARU was formed, but Eugene Debs and Grover Cleveland would eventually confront each other in what one paper would call "the greatest battle between labor and capital that has ever been waged in the United States."

———

By the time the House voted to repeal the Silver Purchase Act on August 28, pro-silver senators knew they probably didn't have enough votes to stave off repeal if the bill reached the Senate floor. So they hoped to kill it before it got there, in the eleven-member Finance Committee, where Chairman Daniel Voorhees would cast the deciding vote. Voorhees was the Indiana senator who generally supported the silver cause but who, in exchange for control of patronage in his home state, had promised President Cleveland that he would "recognize and justify, as far as may be in my power, the generous confidence and friendly regard you have extended to me."

But if Voorhees betrayed them, the silverites had another, more drastic option. Unlike the House, the Senate had a tradition of "unlimited debate" that the silverites intended to exploit to the fullest if necessary. In other words, they would filibuster. Today a vote of three-fifths of the senators—sixty—invokes cloture, bringing debate to an end; but at the time, there was no cloture rule in the Senate. Each senator was allowed to speak as long as he wished. As long as the silverites could keep talking, the Senate couldn't vote on repeal. One pro-silver senator predicted he and his like-minded colleagues could hold out for six months—which, of course, would be six more months during which the Treasury would be required to purchase 4.5 million ounces of silver. Senator Isham Harris of Tennessee promised to filibuster "till Hell froze over."

The silverites also had a valuable ally in Vice President Adlai Stevenson, who, as president of the Senate, would preside over the debate. If, as expected, he was sympathetic to the silverites, the filibuster theoretically could last indefinitely. At the very least it might force the goldbugs to compromise.

Hanging over the debate was the specter of President Cleveland's demise. If, as E. J. Edwards had just reported, Cleveland's body had been invaded by "that dread and mysterious enemy which physicians scarcely dare to name," it was possible that Adlai Stevenson would ascend to the presidency, in which case the special session would be rendered moot. Stevenson would never sign a repeal bill.

The silverites lost the first round when the Finance Committee voted to send the bill to the full Senate for consideration. As expected the vote was six to five, with Daniel Voorhees casting the decisive vote. He had kept his promise to the president. For that, the silverites vilified Voorhees as a Judas, though the senator, unlike the apostle, did it for gold, not silver.

The Senate debate over repeal would eventually fill five volumes of the *Congressional Record* with twenty million words, which, if written on a single line, would have stretched the sixteen hundred miles from Wall Street to Colorado's silver country. Emotions ran high. Colorado senator Henry Teller broke down in tears at his desk. On several occasions opposing senators nearly came to blows. During an especially longwinded speech, Nebraska senator William Allen was interrupted by Senator George Frisbie Hoar of Massachusetts.

"The Senator from Nebraska said a while ago that there was no overproduction," Hoar said. "Does he not regard his speech as an instance of overproduction?"

Allen apparently couldn't take a joke. "The question is too insulting for me to answer!" he thundered in reply.

Though outnumbered, the silverites were entrenched and refused to allow the debate to end. It became an endurance contest. During one stretch, the Senate was in session for thirty-eight continuous hours. With a sympathetic Adlai Stevenson wielding the gavel, William Allen managed to speak for fifteen hours straight at one point, though he spent much of that time reading books aloud.

The debate also exposed how fundamentally undemocratic the United States Senate can be. The four senators from Colorado and Nevada represented fewer than five hundred thousand people, while New York's two senators represented six million. The *New York World* wondered how it was democratic for one-sixtieth of the population to thwart the will of the other fifty-nine sixtieths. It was an exaggeration, but the paper had a point. When an official from the New Mexico Territory met with President Cleveland to make the case for statehood, the president was unmoved. "If that Territory be admitted," Cleveland said, "it will bring to the Senate two more free silver Senators."

On Saturday, October 21, a weary group of Democratic senators from both sides of the issue proposed a compromise: the Silver Purchase Act would be repealed, but not until July 1, 1894, more than eight months hence. They presented the proposal to Cleveland, who angrily rejected it. He insisted he would only sign a bill that repealed the act entirely and immediately. There would be no compromise.

Cleveland's stand broke the filibuster. The silverites realized their cause was hopeless, and their ranks began to crack. On the morning of Tuesday, October 24, Fred Dubois, a pro-silver senator from Idaho, glumly told reporters: "The jig is up." One newspaper facetiously reported that Isham Harris, the senator who had promised to filibuster until hell froze over, "had his skates on ready to take advantage of the freshly formed sheet of ice."

That afternoon, Senator John P. Jones of Nevada took the floor and quietly announced to a hushed chamber that "it is not the intention of anyone connected with this discussion to prolong it any more than is necessary to give his views fully to the Senate and to the people of the country." It was the white flag of surrender.

The final vote would not come until October 30: forty-eight to thirty-seven in favor of repeal. The Senate filibuster had lasted sixty-two days. It still stands as one of the longest filibusters in Senate history, eclipsing even the fifty-seven-day filibuster against the Civil Rights Act of 1964.

For procedural reasons, the bill went back to the House, which formally ratified it two days later, on November 1. The bill was then rushed to the White House. Cleveland, still very much alive and well, signed it into law at four thirty that afternoon by simply writing in the lower left corner of the document, "Approved, Nov. 1, 1893. Grover Cleveland." The bill was law. The Silver Purchase Act was repealed.

"The outcome of the fight is a great personal victory for President Cleveland," the *Washington Post* said.

The battle had been won.

Alas, the war would not be. The repeal of the Silver Purchase Act did not, as Grover had hoped, restore confidence in the economy. It was too little, too late. The panic did not end. By one estimate, unemployment stayed above 10 percent for the next five years—the longest stretch of double-digit unemployment outside the Great Depression. What was needed was a radical overhaul of the nation's financial system, including aggressive governmental oversight. A commission investigating labor unrest at the time faulted the government "for not adequately controlling monopolies and corporations, and for failing to reasonably protect the rights of labor to redress its wrongs." A rudimentary public welfare program would have been helpful as well.

In other words, what was needed was the kind of interventionist "paternalism" that Grover instinctively abhorred.

Although Dr. Bryant had pronounced Grover "all healed" on September 1, in some ways the president never fully recovered from his ordeal

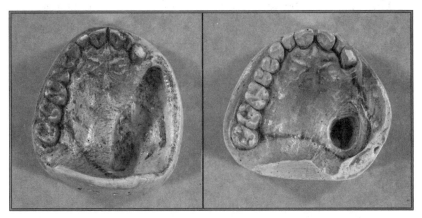

These casts of Grover's mouth were made by the dentist Kasson Gibson shortly after the operation in 1893 (left) and again in 1897 (right).The shrinking of the operative defect is indicative of the remarkable healing that occurred in that time. NEW YORK ACADEMY OF MEDICINE LIBRARY

on the *Oneida*. It is true that the wound inside his mouth healed with noteworthy rapidity. In 1897, the dentist Kasson Gibson made another cast of Grover's mouth to fashion a new prosthesis. It showed the defect had shrunk from 63.5-by-20.6 millimeters to 17.5-by-11.1 millimeters in the four years since the operation, a reduction that many doctors today find remarkable.

Yet Grover was never quite the same after the operation. He was thinner, and he tired easily. He complained of a constant earache—possibly because his uvula was displaced as a result of the operation. And his already legendarily short temper grew even shorter. Cleveland's biographers have tended to minimize the impact of the operation on the remainder of his presidency, but it may have affected his judgment. Before the operation he made decisions only after careful deliberation. Afterward he acted much more rashly. His private secretary, Robert O'Brien, believed the operation "very greatly influenced Mr. Cleveland's mentality."

"He was a considerably different man in the years that followed," O'Brien said. "He worried more easily and was more sensitive. It was a disturbing period in our economic history and he was disturbed by it."

According to O'Brien, after the operation Grover had a tendency to "dismiss things that troubled him rather peremptorily." As an example of this disposition, O'Brien cited an incident involving a group of suffragist women who were holding a conference in Washington. Some of the women requested a meeting with the First Lady. Frances passed the letter along to O'Brien, instructing him to ask the president how it should be answered. Grover, it should be noted, was not sympathetic to the cause of woman's suffrage. (Neither was Frances, for that matter.) When O'Brien approached the president, Grover "did little more than shake his head." All he said was: "Do not receive them." When Grover's name was mentioned at the conference, there was a storm of hisses that only Susan B. Anthony herself was able to calm.

Grover's tendency to dismiss troubling things peremptorily may have also exhibited itself in far more serious ways—as when he clashed with Eugene V. Debs and the American Railway Union.

In the summer of 1893, George Pullman began laying off workers and cutting wages at his factory outside Chicago. Pullman's Palace Car Company manufactured luxury rail cars. Its workers were compelled to live in a town called Pullman, which the company owned lock, stock, and barrel. The workers paid their rents to Pullman. They bought their groceries, water, and gas from Pullman. To some it was a "model town." To others it was more like a feudal system out of the Middle Ages, an example of "corporate despotism."

Between July 1893 and July 1894, the Pullman Company reduced its workforce from fifty-five hundred to thirty-three hundred, and the remaining workers saw their pay reduced by as much as 50 percent. Yet dividends still rose from $2.52 million to $2.88 million. And Pullman refused to lower the rents in the company town, even though they were as much as 25 percent higher than in neighboring communities. Lowering the rents, Pullman later said, "would have amounted to a gift of money to these men; it was simply a matter of business." By early 1894, many workers were on starvation wages. It was estimated that, after the rent and other fees were paid, a typical worker had just six dollars a week left over to feed and clothe his family. Some had mere pennies.

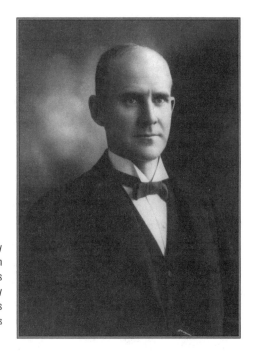

Eugene V. Debs led the American Railway Union's strike against the Pullman Company in 1894. President Cleveland's heavy-handed reaction to the strike may have been due to the aftereffects of his operation. LIBRARY OF CONGRESS

Disgruntled Pullman workers turned to Eugene Debs and his new American Railway Union for help. About four thousand of them joined the ARU. In May 1894, a delegation of workers called on Pullman and asked him to either raise wages or reduce rents. Pullman refused. And for good measure he fired three members of the delegation. The ARU responded with an ultimatum to Pullman: accept arbitration for our grievances, or we will strike. Again, Pullman refused.

The strike began on June 26. ARU members nationwide refused to work on any train with a Pullman car. As Debs recalled,

> The switchmen, in the first place, refused to attach a Pullman car to a train, and that is where the trouble began; and then, when a switchman would be discharged for that, they would all simultaneously quit, as they had agreed to do. One department

after another was involved until the Illinois Central was paralyzed,
and the Rock Island and other roads in their turn.

Within days, the strike spread to twenty-seven states and territories.
More than one hundred thousand workers walked off the job. Rail traffic between Chicago and the West Coast was paralyzed. A labor revolt
of this magnitude was unprecedented in American history. And it was
also noteworthy for its lack of violence. On orders from Debs, the strikers were to remain orderly.

The railroads were suffering incalculable losses, but they were intent
on not only breaking the strike but on wiping out the ARU altogether.
A federal investigation later concluded that the railroads were "determined to crush the strike rather than accept any peaceable solution
through conciliation, arbitration, otherwise." It would be, in the words
of historian Allan Nevins, "a struggle to the death."

But in this struggle the railroads had an important ally: Attorney
General Richard Olney. Before joining the Cleveland administration,
Olney had worked for many years as an attorney for various railroads,
including the New York Central and the Santa Fe. He could hardly be
expected to be neutral in the dispute. And he wasn't.

Olney was known for his belligerence. His fits of rage made his sub-
ordinates in the Justice Department tremble. After his daughter had the
temerity to marry a dentist—imagine!—he barred the couple from his
home. The Pullman strike, Olney decided, must be "smashed," and he
would smash it with characteristic ruthlessness.

The strike had interrupted mail delivery, which gave Olney the pre-
text he needed. Debs and three other union leaders were arrested for
"conspiracy to interfere with interstate commerce," and Olney obtained
an injunction against the strikers. Claiming the country was on "the
ragged edge of anarchy," the attorney general also convinced President
Cleveland to send federal troops to Chicago, ostensibly to restore order
and protect the mail.

Not that Grover needed much convincing. "If it takes the entire
army and navy of the United States to deliver a postal card in Chicago,"

the president bellowed, "that card will be delivered." On July 4, 1894, thousands of troops from Fort Sheridan began marching into the city. Many Chicagoans assumed they were there for an Independence Day celebration. So much for the ragged edge of anarchy. Only after the troops arrived did the strike turn violent. Twelve people would die in clashes with the soldiers.

Illinois governor John Peter Altgeld was a Democrat, and he had campaigned hard for Cleveland in 1892. But in a withering twelve-hundred-word telegram, Altgeld excoriated the president for sending in the troops:

> Surely the facts have not been correctly presented to you in this case or you would not have taken the step; for it is entirely unnecessary and, it seems to me, unjustifiable. Waiving all questions of courtesy, I will say that the State of Illinois is not only able to take care of itself, but it stands ready today to furnish the Federal Government any assistance it may need elsewhere. . . .
>
> As Governor of the State of Illinois, I protest against this, and ask for the immediate withdrawal of the Federal troops from active duty in this State.

Grover responded curtly that "the presence of Federal troops in the city of Chicago was deemed not only proper, but necessary" to end "obstruction of the mails." When Altgeld replied with another long telegram demanding the withdrawal of the troops, Grover hit his limit. "[I]t seems to me," he wired the governor, "that in this hour of danger and public distress, discussion may well give way to active efforts on the part of all in authority to restore obedience to law and to protect life and property."

With Debs and other union leaders in jail, and federal troops in the streets, the Pullman strike collapsed. Debs was never convicted of the conspiracy charge, but he was found guilty of contempt for violating the injunction and sentenced to six months in prison. The American Railway Union collapsed, too. Its last national meeting was held in 1897.

Debs emerged from prison thoroughly radicalized. He helped organize the Socialist Party of America and was its presidential candidate five times. In the 1920 presidential election he received more than nine hundred thousand votes. Six years later he died at the age of sixty-one.

The Pullman strike coincided with the first anniversary of Grover's secret operation, and it may have been one of those troubling things that he was now inclined to dismiss peremptorily. Before the operation, would he have acceded so readily to Olney's desire to smash the strike? Would he have ordered the army into Chicago? Would he have rejected so blithely the objections of Governor Altgeld? The answers are unknowable, of course, but even Cleveland's most sympathetic biographers believe he overreacted. The injunction, writes Allan Nevins, was "improperly drastic," and "the order to send the troops into Chicago was premature." In *The Presidencies of Grover Cleveland*, Richard E. Welch Jr. goes even further. "Cleveland," Welch writes, "permitted the judicial and the military force of the federal government to be used in a manner that was of exclusive benefit to one party in a labor-management dispute."

The repeal of the Silver Purchase Act did not stanch the flow of gold from the U.S. Treasury, and by January 1894 the reserve had shrunk to just $65 million. Twice that year the government issued bonds to replenish the reserve, but the scheme backfired. Most people paid for the bonds by cashing in their silver certificates for gold. "Peter paid Paul," one observer noted, "and the gold reserve was not increased in the process." On January 1, 1895, the reserve stood at just $45 million. Desperate, Grover arranged for another bond sale. Only this time the bonds would be purchased by a syndicate that promised to pay $65 million in gold for them. The syndicate was headed by the financier J. P. Morgan, whom Grover had come to know while living in New York between his presidential terms. The two men met at the White House on the night of February 7, 1895, to hash out the transaction. Grover later insisted that Morgan was acting out of "clear-sighted, far-seeing patriotism." "He was not looking for a personal bargain," Grover told an interviewer, "but sat there, a great patriotic banker, concerting with me and my advisers measures to avert peril, determined to do his best in a severe and trying crisis." The great patriotic banker made a killing on the deal. The syndicate turned around and sold the bonds on the open market for a profit of $7 million.

In a sense, the deal worked. By June the Treasury's gold reserve had once again topped the symbolically important $100 million mark. But the "Cleveland Depression," as many had taken to calling it, still did not end, and Cleveland paid a steep political price for his bargain with Morgan. Coming just seven months after his heavy-handed intervention in the Pullman strike, the Morgan bond deal reinforced a growing perception that Grover Cleveland was merely a tool of rapacious capitalists—many of whom were now among his closest friends.

Grover never seriously considered running for a third term in 1896. He felt bound by precedent. No president had ever served more than two terms. He was also exhausted. He'd lost sixty pounds, and he believed he might never recover from "the mental twist and wrench" of his second term. He lived in fear that the cancer that had been removed on the *Oneida* would someday return, a fear compounded by the fact that he was a fifty-nine-year-old father of three small children—a third daughter, Marion, had been born at Gray Gables in 1895.

Grover never would have won reelection anyway. Hundreds of thousands of destitute and hungry Americans blamed him for the depression and reviled him for his seeming indifference to their suffering. A nasty joke made the rounds: Grover comes upon a starving man eating grass in front of the White House and helpfully advises the man to go around to the backyard because the grass is taller there. Few presidents have left office as unpopular as Grover Cleveland. He was probably the most despised man in America. He received so many threatening letters that the number of police officers assigned to guard the White House was increased from two to twenty-seven. This further outraged many Americans, who saw no reason why their president should be surrounded by bodyguards like a king.

By 1896 even his own party was repudiating Grover Cleveland. At the Democratic National Convention in Chicago, delegates hurled more insults at Grover than at Republican presidential nominee William McKinley. "You ask us to endorse Cleveland's fidelity," said good old Ben "Pitchfork" Tillman. "In reply, I say he has been faithful unto death—the death of the Democratic Party." Tillman went on to condemn the Cleveland administration as "undemocratic and tyrannical."

The Democrats were hopelessly split between the goldbugs and the silverites. At the convention, the silver prophet William Jennings Bryan roused delegates with a scathing attack on the goldbugs: "Having behind us the producing masses of this nation and the world, supported by the commercial interests, the laboring interests and the toilers everywhere, we will answer their demand for a gold standard by saying to them: You shall not press down upon the brow of labor this crown of thorns; you shall not crucify mankind upon a cross of gold!"

Bryan won the nomination, and the delegates adopted a pro-silver plank by the overwhelming vote of 628 to 301. The Democratic Party was now officially in the hands of the silverites, who would continue to fight for bimetallism. The party would remain fractured for a generation.

Grover followed the convention from Gray Gables, where he was enjoying "first-rate" fishing on Buzzards Bay. He was not enjoying the updates coming from Chicago, however. Grover's contempt for William Jennings Bryan was plain. He believed Bryan was a demagogue. "I cannot write or speak favorably of Bryanism." Grover wrote a friend. "I do not regard it as Democracy." To Grover, Bryan and his followers were "haphazard blunderbuss shooters."

Even in these trying times, however, Grover managed to maintain a modicum of good humor. On June 16, 1896, he wrote a letter to Kasson Gibson, the dentist who had fashioned his oral prosthesis. "This morning about an hour ago," Grover wrote, "there came out of a tooth in my right under jaw, next to the dead tooth you fixed up, a piece of gold about the size of a pea. This indicates how completely I have been on the gold standard."

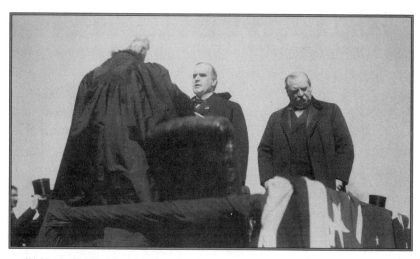

Chief Justice Melville Fuller administers the oath of office to William McKinley while outgoing president Grover Cleveland looks on, March 4, 1897. Cleveland was suffering from a severe case of gout that day and was barely able to stand. LIBRARY OF CONGRESS

After the convention, goldbug Democrats nominated their own candidate for president, Illinois senator John Palmer. Grover voted for Palmer, and although McKinley easily won the election, Grover was not entirely displeased, for McKinley was a goldbug.

While he was now free of cancer—for the time being, at least—Grover continued to be plagued by another infirmity with which he had struggled for years. On Inauguration Day 1897—Grover's last day in office—his gout was so painful that he could barely stand. When McKinley called on him at the White House, Grover was limping heavily, and his foot was bandaged. As it had been four years earlier, the meeting of the incoming and outgoing presidents was amicable. Grover found McKinley to be "an honest, sincere, and serious man." The two men shared a drink of rye whiskey before riding together in an open carriage to the ceremonies at the Capitol. The weather was clear and mild—what used to be called Cleveland weather.

In the summer of 1897, less than six months after Grover left office, ships began arriving in West Coast ports with fantastic tales of huge gold deposits along the Klondike River in the Yukon Territory of northwestern Canada. Gold nuggets were said to be lying on the ground, just waiting to be collected by anyone willing to make the arduous journey to the region. Many were willing. Some forty thousand prospectors descended on the Klondike in the biggest gold rush in history. Many were motivated by sheer desperation. Eventually the Klondike would yield more than ten million ounces of gold, much of which found its way to the U.S. Treasury. This dramatically increased the country's money supply, which, ironically, is exactly what the silverites had hoped to achieve all along. The Spanish-American War gave the economy another boost, and by 1900 the Cleveland Depression, which had begun with the Panic of 1893, had finally lifted.

In 1900 Congress officially made gold the single standard of currency in the United States—though, owing to the Treasury's vast silver reserves (accumulated partly as a result of the Silver Purchase Act), silver certificates continued to be issued and redeemable until the 1960s. FDR took the country off the gold standard in 1933, although technically the value of a dollar remained tied to gold through international treaties until 1971.

On the recommendation of a friend named Andrew West, Grover retired to Princeton, New Jersey. He and Frances bought a big house, which they christened Westland in honor of their friend. The Clevelands had two more children in Princeton, both boys: Richard was born in 1897 and Francis in 1903.

Grover had saved a small fortune by the time he left office, perhaps $300,000, but his advancing age and expanding family caused him to worry constantly about money. Ex-presidents did not receive pensions at the time, and Grover was anxious to "make everything snug" for his family before he died. He wrote a series of articles for the *Saturday Evening Post* and several other publications. For some he was paid as much as $2,500. Friends begged him to write his autobiography, but he demurred. "I want my wife and children to love me now and hereafter to proudly honor my memory," he wrote one friend. "They will have my autobiography written on their hearts where every day they may turn the pages and read it."

On January 2, 1904, the Clevelands' eldest child, twelve-year-old Ruth, came down with tonsillitis. On January 6 she was diagnosed with diphtheria. The next day she was dead. "It seems to me I mourn our darling Ruth's death more and more," Grover wrote on January 15. "So

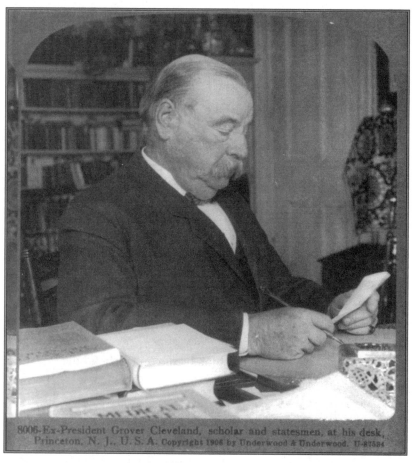

Grover working at his home in Princeton, New Jersey, 1906. In his retirement, the former president became a beloved figure in the town. The university awarded him an honorary degree, and students celebrated football victories by parading to his house. LIBRARY OF CONGRESS

much of the time I can only think of her as dead, not joyfully living in heaven." Grover and Frances could not bear the thought of returning to Gray Gables without Ruth, so they leased the property. The building was eventually turned into an inn and became a popular local restaurant. It was destroyed by arson in 1973. The crime is still unsolved.

Much to his surprise and delight, Grover became a popular figure in Princeton. The university awarded him an honorary degree. Students serenaded him on his birthday, and football victories were celebrated with a parade to Westland, where Grover would appear on the porch to lead the school cheer. For Grover, who had been forced to forego college in order to support his family, his time in Princeton was deeply satisfying.

In 1901 Grover was appointed a trustee of the university. It was in this position that he came to intimately know—and occasionally clash with—the university's president, a sickly history professor named Woodrow Wilson. In 1912, Wilson would become the first Democrat elected president since Grover.

In retirement Grover's frosty relations with the press did not thaw. Once, when an aggressive reporter pressed him for his position on a particularly contentious issue, Grover declared, "That, sir, is a matter of too great importance to discuss in a five-minute interview, now rapidly drawing to its close." He was an elder statesman now, but not all the rough edges from his salad days in Buffalo had been made smooth. He still "trimmed" his cigars by biting off the ends.

In the spring of 1908 Grover's health began to fail precipitously. He complained of stomach pains and was bedridden. At 8:40 on the morning of June 24, he died in his bed at Westland. He was seventy-one. Frances was at his side. His last words were: "I have tried so hard to do right." Naturally, none of his lengthy obituaries mentioned the operation on the *Oneida* in 1893. It was still a closely guarded secret.

Grover Cleveland was buried in Princeton Cemetery on June 26. His tombstone does not mention the fact that he was twice president of the United States. His grave is just a short walk away from the grave of the eighteenth-century theologian Jonathan Edwards—a collateral ancestor of E. J. Edwards.

Grover survived fifteen years after his secret surgery. The cancer in his mouth never recurred, a fact that pleased Dr. William Williams Keen immensely. "That he should have survived after the removal of a sarcoma of the jaw without local recurrence for so unusually long a period was a great satisfaction to Dr. Bryant and his colleagues." However, the exact nature of Grover's final illness and the cause of his death are unclear. Biographer Allan Nevins believed Grover "was in the grip of gastro-intestinal disease complicated by ailments of the heart and kidneys." On his death certificate the cause is listed as "heart failure complicated with pulmonary thrombosis and edema." But Dr. John Erdmann, who had assisted in the operation on the *Oneida*, later told an interviewer that he believed Grover died from "an intestinal obstruction" and that a postmortem examination revealed "extensive carcinoma . . . in the intestines." The records from this examination have been lost, but if Grover did indeed have intestinal cancer, an interesting question is raised: Were the oral tumor and the intestinal tumor related? In other words, had the oral cancer finally metastasized as Grover long feared?

The answer, it turned out, was in a small glass jar.

Despite the harsh treatment he received at the hands of Grover's minions, E. J. Edwards did not hold it against the president. In November 1893, just months after reporting what really happened on the *Oneida*, Edwards published a long and flattering profile of Grover in *McClure's Magazine*. Ironically, Edwards described the essence of Grover's character as "the courage of truth" and his only political fault as "honesty."

Edwards continued cranking out twenty-five-hundred-word columns for the *Press* six days a week, and in 1894 he scored another brilliant beat, one for which he would once again be vilified—and, this time, nearly thrown in jail. The affair became known as the Sugar Trust scandal.

At the time, the U.S. sugar industry was controlled by a single entity formally known as the American Sugar Refining Company, but better known simply as the Sugar Trust. Styled along the lines of the other great trusts, including Rockefeller's Standard Oil, the Sugar Trust was a coalition of twenty-four sugar refiners that had banded together in 1887 in hopes of "lessening the expenses of production, culling . . . useless employees, and preventing overproduction." It was, in other words, a monopoly. By 1893 the Sugar Trust controlled the industry from the cane fields to the coffee cup. As the world's largest buyer of raw sugarcane, it dictated prices. Planters had to either accept the trust's offer or "eat their sugar." Retail prices were likewise fixed. It was estimated the Sugar Trust raked in as much as $35 million in profit annually. "Other trusts there are as illegal and as wicked in intention," the *New York World* wrote, "but none so successfully rapacious, so completely in control of a product necessary to civilized men in all stations, or so merciless in abusing that control."

As the owner of the largest refinery in the trust, Henry O. Havemeyer had more or less total control of the enterprise. Havemeyer was the epitome of the nineteenth-century robber baron. While the country was sinking into depression in 1893, he was said to be "earning" $2 million a month. He and his second wife were prolific and relatively tasteful art collectors. Hundreds of their pieces would eventually be donated to the Metropolitan Museum of Art, including works by Degas, Monet, and Rembrandt. (Evidently, however, Henry's business savvy failed him in the art world. Twelve of his fifteen Renoirs turned out to be forgeries.)

The robber barons were a loathsome bunch, but few were loathed as passionately as Henry Havemeyer. In the treatment of his workers he made George Pullman look like Dorothea Dix. In the summer of 1892, twenty-four firemen who stoked the massive boilers in Havemeyer's refinery died from injuries and illnesses caused by the scalding heat in the boiler room. The following June, the firemen went on strike. Their only demand was that the length of the workday be decreased from twelve hours to eight hours during the summer. Havemeyer refused, and replaced the striking workers.

Clearly Henry Havemeyer was not a man to be trifled with, but E. J. Edwards did just that—and managed to antagonize the U.S. Senate in the process.

In his Holland letter in the *Press* on May 14, 1894, Edwards reported that Havemeyer had met with Grover in the summer of 1892 to discuss the "interests" of the Sugar Trust. According to Edwards, the trust "contributed the magnificent sum of $500,000" to the Democratic campaign that fall, with the understanding that the party would not endorse legislation "antagonistic" to the trust. At the time, a half-cent tariff was imposed on every pound of refined sugar imported into the United States. But this was not a "revenue" tariff that raised money for the government. It was a "differential" tariff that was paid directly to the Sugar Trust. It was, in other words, a government handout that amounted to roughly $20 million a year. Naturally, Havemeyer was eager to keep this spigot open. As he liked to say, "The tariff is the mother of trusts."

In the fall of 1893, however, a bill that would have entirely eliminated the sugar tariff was passed by the House and referred to the Senate Finance Committee. The following February the Democratic members of that committee were meeting informally when, quite unexpectedly, Treasury Secretary John Carlisle entered the room. "He went secretly and came away secretly," Edwards wrote.

> His visit was supposed to be a confidential one. . . . They looked upon him as speaking, not so much for Mr. Carlisle, as for the administration. He did not say that he came from the President, but when he had finished making his astonishing statement, not one of those who heard him doubted that he had come from the President and was echoing the President's wishes, and giving emphasis to them by an earnest, and for him, excited manner. What he said is quoted from remembrance, but it is substantially accurate, as it was reported by one who heard it. He said:
>
> "Gentlemen, there is one thing that I am bound to say to you as earnestly and impressively as I can do it, and I speak to you as a Democrat to Democrats. No party or the representatives of no

party can afford to ignore honorable obligations. I want to say to
you that there seems to be danger that this is going to be done.
Gentlemen associated with the sugar refining interests (I may tell
you perhaps what you do not know) subscribed to the campaign
several hundred thousand dollars and at a time when money was
urgently needed. I tell you that it would be wrong, it would be
infamous, after having accepted that important contribution, given
at a time when it was imperatively needed, for the Democratic
party now to turn around and strike down the men who gave it. It
must not be done. I trust that you will prepare an amendment to
the bill which will be reasonable and in some measure satisfactory
to these interests."

That, in substance, was the plea of Secretary Carlisle to
the members of the Finance Committee that they respect the
obligations entered into by the national campaign committee and
the personal representatives of Mr. Cleveland in 1892.

The final version of the bill included a tariff that would result in an
annual windfall of $15 million for the Sugar Trust—$5 million less than
it had received under the old tariff, but, apparently, enough to satisfy
Havemeyer. Cleveland, who professed to be opposed to tariffs, allowed
the bill to become law without his signature.

Edwards also reported that at least two senators had purchased large
amounts of Sugar Trust stock after the Finance Committee had decided
to restore the tariff but before its decision was made public. One of
the senators, Edwards estimated, had made $500,000 "by reason of his
good fortune in procuring inside knowledge."

Edwards's accusations were explosive. Indignant senators, their
honor offended, demanded an investigation. On May 17, 1894, just
three days after the story was published, the Senate passed a resolution
creating a special committee to look into Edwards's allegations. A few
days after that, Edwards received a telegram: "You are requested to
appear before the committee. Do you accept this as a legal summons?
Answer."

Edwards appeared before the committee on May 24. It quickly became apparent that the panel was less interested in ascertaining the veracity of his account than in finding out who squealed. During the proceedings, the committee's chairman, Delaware senator George Gray asked Edwards point-blank: "Who was your informant?" Edwards responded,

> That, I suppose, I shall have to decline to answer. I do it with the utmost respect to the committee and the Senate. The information was given to me under obligations of the highest confidentiality by the one who entailed that obligation, so that I do not feel at liberty to reveal his name.

That would not do. Nebraska senator William Allen picked up the cudgel for the committee.

> Senator Allen: Was the man a member of Congress?
>
> Mr. Edwards: I suppose that is in the nature of cross-examination tending to get me to disclose. But I will say that he is not a member of Congress.
>
> Senator Allen: Was he a clerk in the employ of the Government?
>
> Mr. Edwards: I ought to draw the line at that question, and I decline to answer it. I do it with respect.
>
> Senator Allen: You understand, you have no right to secrete the name of any such person when you are called upon in an examination of this kind. We have a right to demand the name of you. The only shield you have here is you are at liberty not to testify on any subject that would subject you to a criminal prosecution. If the statement does not criminate you under the law, you can not conceal that name. Do you understand that to be the case?
>
> Mr. Edwards: I do not.
>
> Senator Allen: That is true. Under those circumstances, do you still refuse to disclose the man's name?
>
> Mr. Edwards: I think I should like to get the opinion of counsel

about that. My sense of honor in regard to that gentleman is so delicate; I want to do what is right; I want to meet my obligation with perfect freedom.

The committee adjourned to allow Edwards to fetch his lawyer. When testimony resumed, Edwards still refused to identify his source. His lawyer, Abram Dittenhoefer, argued that the senators were seeking information that was "utterly unnecessary."

> It is unimportant for the committee, for the purpose of arriving at the truth of the alleged charge, to ascertain who informed Mr. Edwards. The question before the committee is whether the charge is true or false, not who gave the information. . . .
>
> Lastly, being a newspaper man, the witness is under honorable obligations not to disclose the source of his information, because if he violated that obligation of honor it would degrade him in the estimation, not only of members of his own profession, but of the entire community.

The committee was not moved by Dittenhoefer's argument. "The objections made by the witness under the instructions of his counsel were overruled," the transcript of the hearing curtly notes, "and the witness was directed to answer." Still, Edwards refused, and on May 29 the Senate passed a resolution charging him with contempt and ordering his arrest. It was a serious charge. If convicted, Edwards could be jailed. And the threat was real. In 1871 the Senate had jailed two *New York Tribune* reporters who refused to identify a source.

After Edwards testified, the special committee summoned the Democratic members of the Finance Committee to appear. To a man, the senators denied what Edwards had reported, and for the second time in less than a year his name was dragged through the mud.

> George Vest of Missouri: "Nothing of that kind occurred in our committee."

Daniel Voorhees of Indiana: "There is not a single word of truth in the article—not a word."

Roger Mills of Texas: "I know nothing on earth about it."

And so on. Treasury Secretary Carlisle also testified that Edwards's report was "absolutely false."

His old nemesis, *Philadelphia Times* publisher Alexander McClure, was only too happy to pile on. "He published columns of compiled gossip and scandal about Senators and other government officials, and the Sugar Trust," the *Times* said of Edwards in an editorial,

> [B]ut he skulks behind innuendoes and indefinite generalities as to individuals, and when called upon to allow the Senate to vindicate itself by naming its accusers, so that they could be brought face to face, he seals his lips and calls his scandals privileged communications made to him in confidence.
>
> This is simply a burlesque on journalistic dignity and decency, and it is the duty of Mr. Edwards either to give the Senate information to enable it to probe the truth of the gossip, or to confess that his publication was a sensational and unjustifiable scandal.

On August 2, the special committee issued its findings. Citing no more evidence than the testimony of the senators under suspicion, the report exonerated them and concluded that Edwards's allegations were "without foundation in fact and utterly untrue." The report went on to say, "The conduct of Mr. Edwards in making and publishing so specific and serious a charge against public men, and one affecting their discharge of high public duties, upon no personal knowledge, and upon no information, the source of which he is willing to disclose, calls for serious reprobation."

Edwards was allowed to remain free until he had his day in court, which came on Friday, June 18, 1897, more than three years after he had published the Sugar Trust story.

It was not a long day. After listening to testimony from just three witnesses, including the special committee's chairman, George Gray, a District of Columbia judge ruled that the telegram the committee had sent to Edwards was not a legal summons. Therefore, Edwards could not be held in contempt. Besides, the judge added, the questions Edwards had refused to answer "were not pertinent to the inquiry." The judge ordered the jury to render a verdict of not guilty, which was done.

Although Edwards had been acquitted on a technicality, the court was clearly sympathetic to the argument that he should not be forced to identify his source. In some ways it was a landmark case. Edwards's lawyer, Abram Dittenhoefer, considered the verdict "a great victory for the newspaper profession." In an editorial, Edwards's paper agreed. It was only a matter of time, the *Press* wrote, before the law would fully recognize "the privilege of journalism in protecting confidential sources of information."

> The principle is just in reason and in practice. It is vital to liberty and it does not conduce to license. It is inherent in the very conditions of modern journalism. It is just as essential in the operation of modern social and public forces as any power of Congress itself, and the time will come when it will be declared from the bench as it will be recognized in legislative halls.

That time, alas, has not yet come. Reporters can still be jailed for protecting their sources. In 2005, Judith Miller of the *New York Times* spent eighty-five days behind bars for refusing to tell a grand jury how she learned the identity of CIA agent Valerie Plame.

Edwards's account of the Sugar Trust scandal was corroborated by another reporter at the time. John Shriver of the *New York Mail and Express* said he learned of the secret meeting between Treasury Secretary Carlisle and the Democratic members of the Finance Committee from a member of Congress whom he refused to identify.

Like Edwards, Shriver was charged with contempt for refusing to cooperate with the special committee investigating the scandal. Three other people, including Henry Havemeyer, were also charged. All but one were acquitted. Elverton Chapman, a New York stockbroker who refused to identify his clients, was found guilty and served thirty days in a Washington jail.

In 1900 the Sugar Trust renamed itself after one of its most popular brands and became Domino Sugar. Seven years later, Henry Havemeyer died of heart failure. He was sixty. He left an estate valued at anywhere from $10 million to $40 million ($200 million to $800 million today). The sole beneficiaries were his wife and three children.

E. J. Edwards's career would continue well into the third decade of the twentieth century, but he would always remain a man of the nineteenth. He never abandoned his thick walrus moustache, even after it had long passed out of fashion. He adopted the typewriter only grudgingly and only at the insistence of his considerably younger editors, who were frustrated when his penmanship deteriorated due to cataracts. Later he would dictate his columns to a stenographer.

Edwards continued writing his Holland letters for the *Philadelphia Press* until 1909, when he moved to the *Wall Street Journal*. He was sixty-two at the time, and his new position was less demanding: He was asked to write only three or four columns a week, half his usual output at the *Press*. He also wrote a syndicated column of reminiscences called "New News of Yesterday."

It was a fine career—but one seemingly tainted forever by allegations that he had faked the story about the secret operation on Grover Cleveland.

11

THE TRUTH (AT LAST)

IN THE MONTHS FOLLOWING the operation on the *Oneida*, William Williams Keen went to Washington several times to examine Grover's mouth. "In these visits," Keen recalled, "I usually lunched with the family and saw Mrs. Cleveland and the children, who were charming young girls." Twelve years later, in 1905, Keen twice saw Grover in consultation with Dr. Bryant at Westland, the Cleveland home in Princeton. The former president complained of severe abdominal pain. "Owing to his excessively fat belly walls," Keen wrote, "it was impossible to examine the abdominal viscera with accuracy." Like Dr. Erdmann, Keen suspected the cause was a "malignant growth," but he and Bryant agreed that an operation would be "injudicious" in light of the patient's age and condition.

After Cleveland died, Keen would occasionally run into Frances Cleveland at the office of an eye doctor they both saw. On one occasion, in 1912, Frances was with one of her daughters. Frances said it was an odd coincidence, for only the night before she had told her daughters of the secret operation on their father for the first time.

In 1901, when he was sixty-four, Keen embarked on a two-year trip around the world with two of his daughters. From Philadelphia they headed west to San Francisco, then on to Alaska, Russia, Japan, the Philippines, China, Burma, India, Iran, Turkey, Greece, and Italy. In Manila they had lunch with William Howard Taft, the governor-general of the Philippines. In Burma, Keen broke his clavicle when he was thrown from a horse. In Iran he rather improbably bumped into one of his former students, an Iranian-American named Joseph Shimoon.

As the years passed, laurels were heaped upon Keen. He collected honorary degrees from Northwestern, Edinburgh, and Yale. The Royal College of Surgeons and the American College of Surgeons both made him an honorary fellow. He followed avidly and with awe the seemingly relentless advance of medicine: the discovery of X-rays (1895), a typhoid fever vaccine (1896), the first successful human blood transfusion (1907).

He crossed paths with more presidents, too. When William McKinley was a congressman, Keen performed a minor operation on McKinley's wife, Ida. After McKinley became president, Keen was invited to lunch with the McKinleys at the White House several times. On one occasion, Ida, who was epileptic, had a seizure during the meal. "She trembled rather violently and convulsively all over," Keen remembered. "In an instant, the president rose, threw his napkin over her head and face, and drew her body and head to his breast." The attack subsided after two or three minutes, which, Keen noted, "seemed an hour." Afterward, lunch resumed as if nothing had happened.

Keen would also come to know Taft and Wilson quite well. Taft, whom he'd met in Manila, sent his daughter to Keen for treatment when she was a student at Bryn Mawr. And when Wilson was governor of New Jersey, Keen operated on Wilson's wife and two of their daughters. The operation on one of the children was very dangerous, Keen recalled, as there was a "furious hemorrhage." "Such an emergency brings the surgeon and the family very closely together." His close relations with both men posed a dilemma for Keen in 1912, when Taft and Wilson ran against each other (and Teddy Roosevelt). Before the election, Keen said he would probably vote for Taft "because he has been a very careful and conservative, and yet progressive, president." We cannot know if Keen ever discussed the Cleveland operation with any of the succeeding presidents with whom he became acquainted. But we do know that Wilson, at least, subscribed to Grover's theory that the less the public knew about his health, the better.

In 1907 Keen resigned his chair at Jefferson Medical College. He had taught medicine for forty-one years, and his students numbered more than ten thousand. But he hardly retired. He advocated tirelessly for evolution and vivisection (experimentation on live animals). He continued to write prolifically, authoring papers for professional journals, as well as medical articles for popular magazines like *Ladies' Home Journal* and the *Saturday Evening Post*. (An example of the latter: "Do Warts and Moles Result in Cancer?" Keen thought they might.) He also wrote several books, including one called *Everlasting Life: A Creed and a Speculation*.

As he aged, Keen said his religious views "liberalized," but he clung tenaciously to his Baptist faith. While he may not have eaten cold roast beef every Sunday, Keen wrote that he did not follow the "modern trend of the almost total secularization of the Sabbath, in fact the total neglect of its religious duties and pleasures." "I do not believe that God is so illogical," he wrote late in life. "There *must* be another and a better world. Otherwise, God (or Nature, if one prefers it) would be a monumental bungler."

Apart from a bad case of diverticulitis, and occasional accidents like that broken clavicle, Keen enjoyed remarkably good health. But in January 1916, when he was seventy-nine, he contracted influenza. It was a serious illness. The ensuing pandemic would claim at least fifty million lives worldwide. Keen went to Florida to recuperate, and while he was there he decided to publish an account of the secret operation on Grover Cleveland.

His health failing but his sense of history acute, Keen realized that the story would soon be lost forever if it wasn't published. Nearly all the other players in the drama were now dead. It had been eight years since Grover's passing. Dr. Joseph Bryant, who had always intended to write about the operation, never got around to it before exiting the stage in 1914. Ferdinand Hasbrouck, the much maligned dentist, had died way back in 1904, Dan Lamont in 1905, Edward Janeway in 1911, Robert O'Reilly in 1912. By 1916, just three witnesses to the events on the *Oneida* in July 1893 remained: Keen, Elias Benedict, and John Erdmann, who had been Bryant's young assistant and was now himself an acclaimed surgeon in New York. As Keen later wrote, "I felt it a duty to make the facts a matter of public record before all of us had passed away."

Keen also felt a duty to E. J. Edwards. Keen always regretted how the newspaperman had been so viciously maligned by the *Philadelphia Times*. "His veracity was violently assailed," Keen wrote. "'Fakir' and 'calamity liar' were among the obnoxious epithets applied to him." The entire episode had struck Keen as fundamentally unjust, not to mention unchristian, and it gnawed at his conscience. In 1893, Keen could say nothing—but now he could. By publishing the facts, he said, he would "vindicate Mr. Edwards' character as a truthful correspondent."

Keen was also motivated by a pinch of vanity. The operation and the patient's long postoperative survival stood as signal achievements in his storied career. Yet the full story of those achievements had never been told. Credit should be given, Keen believed, where credit was due. And he, along with the other doctors involved, deserved credit, not just for the successful operation, but also for the small part they played in saving the gold standard.

Before he could write anything, however, Keen deemed it "not only courteous but imperative to ask Mrs. Cleveland's permission." By then, Frances was no longer Mrs. Cleveland; she was Mrs. Preston. In 1913, five years after Grover's death, Frances married a Wells College professor named Thomas J. Preston. She was forty-eight, he was fifty. They had met when he was teaching at Princeton. Frances was the first widow of a president to remarry. (Jacqueline Kennedy is the only other.) One of Frances's biographers has described the marriage as one of "companionship," but it would prove enduring, and Frances would be married to Thomas Preston much longer than she was married to Grover Cleveland.

Keen's health improved, and on February 23 he wrote to Frances. Averring that "as this was a most critical period in the life of the Nation some authoritative record of it ought to be made," he asked for her permission to publish "the facts in the case as a contribution to the political, financial, and surgical history of the country." Five weeks later, on March 30, Frances replied. "I think you are right," she wrote, though she asked to see the manuscript before Keen submitted it for publication. Keen readily agreed and set about finding a suitable outlet for the story. His first choice was the most popular periodical in the country.

Although it claims to be descended from Benjamin Franklin's *Pennsylvania Gazette*, the *Saturday Evening Post* was actually founded in 1821 as a four-page weekly newspaper published every Saturday in Philadelphia. The paper came to be renowned for its political coverage, and developed a national readership. By 1855 it had mutated into a magazine with an impressive weekly circulation of ninety thousand. By 1897, however, circulation had dropped to two thousand, and the *Post* was in danger of folding. In swooped Cyrus Curtis, who bought the magazine for a mere $1,000. Curtis was a robber baron with a philanthropic streak. His fortune was estimated to be as great as J. P. Morgan's, but Curtis gave much of his away to institutions in his adopted hometown of Philadelphia, including the Franklin Institute, Drexel University, and the University of Pennsylvania. In 1899, Curtis hired a thirty-two-year-old Kentuckian named George Horace Lorimer to run the *Post*. The first thing Lorimer did was start putting color illustrations on the cover (one of the illustrators he would hire was a young Norman Rockwell). Then he started filling the magazine with fiction by popular writers like Jack London—*The Call of the Wild* was serialized in the *Post* in 1903. Finally, he added a mix of human interest stories and features on current events. Editorially the *Post* was conservative. Muckrakers found no refuge on its pages. No boats were rocked.

Lorimer's formula proved to be wildly successful. By 1916 the magazine's circulation had exceeded two million, and by the time Lorimer retired in 1936 it would top three million. If W. W. Keen wanted his story to reach the largest audience possible, it would have been impossible to do better than the *Post*. Keen pitched the story to Lorimer, who accepted it immediately. It wasn't every day that the country's most famous surgeon offered to write about a secret operation he had performed on a president of the United States.

It's rather peculiar that Keen chose to publish the story in a mass-market magazine like the *Saturday Evening Post* instead of a medical journal. After all, if the doctors had successfully removed a cancerous tumor with no recurrence of the disease for fifteen years, it was a signal achievement in oncology. And why had the operation been kept under wraps for so long, anyway? Cleveland had been dead for eight years. Why the continuing secrecy? The presidential historian Robert H. Ferrell suspects the doctors had started to have second thoughts about their original diagnosis. In *Ill-Advised: Presidential Health and Public Trust*, Ferrell writes,

> If [Cleveland] had had, as Keen and the others believed, a fast-growing cancer of the mouth, it must have seemed to them that even with their wide-ranging operative procedure . . . the chances of survival for fifteen years would not have been great; most cancers of the mouth, they knew, were likely to recur, if not in the same place, then through metastasis.

Perhaps Keen wanted to avoid the peer review that would attend the publication of the story in a medical journal. Perhaps publication in a medical journal simply would not have satisfied his stated and lofty desire to contribute to the "political, financial, and surgical history of the country." Whatever his motives, Keen plunged into the project with his customary thoroughness. He researched the story for a year. Besides his own notes, he also reviewed the notes of Bryant, Hasbrouck, and O'Reilly. He pored through reams of old newspaper clippings and read several Cleveland biographies. He interviewed Benedict and Erdmann, as well as Kasson Gibson, the dentist who'd fashioned Grover's oral prosthesis. And he began corresponding with E. J. Edwards.

The letters Keen and Edwards exchanged were warm, even friendly. In September 1916 Edwards apologized for a delay in replying to Keen's last letter to him, explaining that he was suffering from "tired nerves." When Keen responded with concern for Edwards's health, the reporter responded, "I appreciate your kindly interest in my health but I am sorry to say that I have been advised to take a spell of complete rest until I am in normal condition." In these exchanges, Edwards told Keen for the first time exactly how he had learned of the operation: Hasbrouck's missed appointment with Carlos MacDonald, Hasbrouck telling MacDonald about the surgery, MacDonald telling Leander Jones, Jones telling Edwards. "It was by pure chance that it was given to me," Edwards explained. "I will say that there was no financial or political motive behind it. Had there been I should not have written the story."

By March 1917, Keen had finished the first draft of his manuscript. He sent a copy to Frances, who complimented him on his effort. "How vividly it brings back to me all the details of that anxious summer," she wrote in a letter to Keen.

The story was published in the September 22, 1917, edition of the *Saturday Evening Post*. On the cover was an illustration of a befuddled doughboy trying to talk to a shy French peasant girl.* Keen's story began on page twenty-four of the 120-page issue. Entitled "The Surgical Operations on President Cleveland in 1893," the article was credited to "W. W. Keen, M.D., LL.D., Emeritus Professor of Surgery, Jefferson Medical College, Philadelphia." It filled three full pages of the oversized periodical and was accompanied by two photographs of Grover taken at his home in Princeton in 1906.

In sixty-five hundred words, Keen adeptly summarizes the turbulent political, financial, and social circumstances surrounding the operation,

---

* The illustrator was J. C. Leyendecker, Norman Rockwell's mentor and, in his time, the most famous illustrator in the country.

though he describes the procedure itself only briefly. The article begins with an homage to E. J. Edwards, noting that his report in the *Philadelphia Press* on August 29, 1893, was "substantially correct, even in most of the details." Keen's version of events is not unbiased, however. He is unapologetic about the secrecy surrounding the operation. "Now, after the lapse of nearly a quarter century," he writes, "it is even more evident than it was at the time that the instant decision of Mr. Cleveland . . . to keep the operation a profound secret was wise, and one may say imperative. What the consequences would have been had it become known at once we can only surmise, and shudder!"

Keen ends the article with a paean to Grover:

> My political principles and convictions differed from his own, but I never questioned his sincerity. He had long had my profound respect, but he gained my affection in the very first hour I passed with him on the deck of the *Oneida*. May this nation be ever blessed with many such noble, fearless citizens!

Despite its name, the *Saturday Evening Post* was usually delivered in the mail on Wednesdays, so E. J. Edwards must have been very impatient for the postman to arrive at his home in Greenwich on Wednesday, September 19. One can imagine him, now nearly seventy and in fragile health, shuffling into his parlor with the magazine in his hand, settling into a comfortable chair, and paging through the advertisements for Cream of Wheat, Campbell's soup, and Firestone tires until he found Keen's article. As he read it, a smile must have come to his face. At long last, he was vindicated.

It also must have occurred to Edwards—and to many other readers—just how profoundly the world had changed since the secret operation on Grover Cleveland. The pages of the *Post* were filled with advertisements for automobiles (a five-passenger Mitchell Junior with a forty-horsepower motor started at $1,250), as well as articles from France, where the American Expeditionary Forces were preparing to join the British and the French on the western front. The Great War was being fought with nimble airplanes that could reach speeds of 130 miles an hour and efficient new machine guns that could mow down the enemy with ghastly efficiency. These advances—if they can be called that—were scarcely imaginable in 1893, when Henry Ford was still tinkering with his first gasoline-powered buggy.

W. W. Keen's *Saturday Evening Post* article caused a sensation among journalists. Not only did it finally solve the mystery of what really took place on the *Oneida* all those years ago; it also vindicated one of their own. A headline in the *Washington Herald* read, "Journalist Who Scooped the World Is Vindicated After Being Branded a 'Faker' for Twenty-five [*sic*] Years."

Edwards was inundated with congratulatory letters and telegrams.

"My congratulations sincere and heartfelt, for the splendid vindication of you contained in the remarkable article by Dr. W. W. Keen," wrote one old colleague. "This article will make up the record that will become traditional of an outstanding newspaper feat."

"I am delighted to have your treatment and report of the Cleveland operation so thoroughly vindicated by such eminent authority as Dr. Keen," wrote Nicholas Murray Butler, the president of Columbia University, which had started a journalism program just five years earlier.

Edwards's old boss, *Philadelphia Press* publisher Charles Emory Smith, had died in 1908, but his successor, Alden March, sent his congratulations on the paper's behalf: "Of course we were all greatly pleased over your vindication by Dr. Keen."

But E. J. would receive no congratulations—and no apologies— from Alexander McClure, the *Philadelphia Times* publisher who had called him a "disgrace to journalism." In 1901, McClure sold the *Times* to Adolph Ochs, the owner of the *New York Times*. McClure retired to his farm outside Philadelphia but lost his fortune just two years later due to "unfortunate investments." Practically penniless, McClure found an unlikely savior: his old nemesis, Charles Emory Smith, the *Philadelphia Press* publisher and prominent Republican. Smith quietly arranged for McClure to be appointed prothonotary, or clerk, of the Pennsylvania Supreme Court, a cushy job that paid a handsome $12,000 a year. On

June 6, 1909, McClure was talking with his family on his front porch when he dropped dead. He was eighty-one.

In 1902, a year after he bought the *Times* from McClure, Adolph Ochs bought another Philadelphia paper, the *Public Ledger*, and merged it with the *Times*, though the new paper was still called the *Public Ledger*. In 1913, Ochs sold the *Public Ledger* to Cyrus Curtis, the publisher of the *Saturday Evening Post*. As a result, technically at least, Curtis owned both the paper that had vilified E. J. Edwards in 1893 and the magazine that vindicated him twenty-four years later. (Another coincidence: in 1920, Curtis would buy Edwards's old paper, the *Philadelphia Press*, and fold it into the *Public Ledger*.)

E. J. Edwards was moved by the outpouring of congratulations that followed the *Post* article. "I cannot tell you how much I appreciate what you wrote of my relation to the operation," Edwards wrote Keen the week after the article was published. "The article must have been widely read as I have received by mail congratulations for the vindication you embodied in the article. When I come to Philadelphia I hope to call upon you and make by hand grasp and face to face greeting the personal acquaintance that will supplement that which has been established by our correspondence."

Keen was gratified. "After suffering in silence for twenty-four years," he wrote of Edwards, "his vindication was now complete."

12

POSTMORTEM

Iᶠ E. J. Eᴅᴡᴀʀᴅs ever made W. W. Keen's acquaintance "by hand grasp and face to face greeting," the event was unrecorded. Edwards was frail in his final years and rarely traveled, though he continued to write columns for the *Wall Street Journal*. In 1918, a year after his vindication, Edwards was paid tribute by the *Washington Herald*, another paper that published his columns over the years: "Under the penname of 'Holland,' this truly remarkable man has presented for more than a quarter of a century an unbiased review of current financial, industrial, commercial, and transportation conditions which has challenged the admiration of the critics and the captains of these various spheres of activity."

In 1920, Edwards attended the Yale Class of 1870's fiftieth reunion. "The years pass on and we go on upon the path our career has already made," he wrote the reunion committee in a rare moment of self-reflection.

I presume the accumulation of words, words, words which identify my various articles . . . would be represented in figures by several million. But it is gratifying to know that much that I have written has been of good influence, for of this I have both the spoken and written proof of many of the leaders in thought and action. My work has not brought many dollars to me, but it has secured for me regard and some influence, such as dollars and cents cannot buy. That is as far as my modesty will permit me to go."

On Thursday, April 17, 1924, E. J. Edwards was dictating to a stenographer in his New York office when he suffered a massive stroke. He was taken to his son's home in Greenwich, where he died eight days later. He was buried in Norwich, Connecticut, on Monday, April 28—the same day his final "Holland" letter was published in the *Wall Street Journal*. His passing elicited little note. The New York and Philadelphia papers ran brief obituaries. None mentioned his woebegone beat in 1893. A short tribute in a small New Hampshire paper said, "He was the kind of man who honored journalism by his connection with it."

In 1918, Dr. William Williams Keen was commissioned an officer in the Medical Reserve Corps of the U.S. Army. Thus he served as a commissioned officer during both the Civil War and World War I, a distinction that may be unique. Keen's role in the latter conflict, however, was purely symbolic. His chief value to the army, he admitted, was as a "stimulating example." Recruiters would implore civilian doctors to volunteer by invoking Keen's vaunted name. "Aren't you husky young fellows going to volunteer," they'd ask, "when Dr. W. W. Keen, almost eighty, was among the first to do so?" According to Keen, "This fetched them, again and again."

Though his military service was token, Keen's medical expertise was still in demand. In August 1921, Keen was vacationing in Bar Harbor, Maine, when he received an urgent telephone call summoning him to Lubec, a town about one hundred miles up the coast. A doctor there,

Eben Bennett, had a patient whose symptoms included a high fever and partial paralysis. Bennett thought it was just a bad cold, but he wanted a second opinion. Keen went to Lubec, and from there he took a boat to an island a few miles offshore to see the patient. The island was called Campobello. The patient's name was Franklin Delano Roosevelt. Keen knew who Roosevelt was, of course: he was a former assistant secretary of the navy, and just the year before he had been the Democratic Party's vice presidential candidate.

Keen must have seemed a godsend to Roosevelt. Harvard had recently awarded the doctor an honorary degree, proclaiming him the "Dean of American Surgery." But Keen was in his eighties now, and virology was not his specialty. He misdiagnosed Roosevelt badly. Keen believed the paralysis in Roosevelt's legs was caused by a blood clot or lesion in the spinal cord. He prescribed vigorous massaging, which Roosevelt found so painful that he demanded another opinion. A doctor from Boston quickly concluded that Roosevelt had contracted polio—and that the massaging was doing much more harm than good. (Medical historians now believe FDR may have actually been suffering not from polio but from a different paralytic illness known as Guillain-Barré syndrome.)

Nevertheless, Keen would remain on good terms with Roosevelt—even after sending him a bill for $600. And, for his part, Roosevelt would go on to orchestrate one of the most fantastic medical masquerades in the annals of the American presidency, passing himself off as able-bodied when he wasn't.

But Keen's reputation was secure. The same year he misdiagnosed FDR, a lavish dinner was held at the Bellevue-Stratford Hotel in Philadelphia to celebrate Keen's eighty-fourth birthday. Speakers lauded him as "one of the greatest American surgeons" and "field marshal of the medical profession." More than two hundred telegrams of congratulations were read, and Keen was presented with a life-size bronze bust of himself.

In an after-dinner speech Keen said, "Long since, I gave up the rather opprobrious phrase 'old age' and have substituted for it the more seductive locution 'accumulated years.' The latter connotes a certain joy in continued acquisition, a sort of pride in adding one annual sparkling jewel after another to an already precious store."

The doctor also prescribed some rules for life. "Mix merry laughter with earnest labor. Always have some as yet unfinished, but not too urgent job waiting just outside your door. Then you will never know ennui. To 'kill time' is murder in the first degree."

W. W. Keen would live another eleven productive years. At ninety-one, he wrote an article for the *Atlantic Monthly* decrying the high cost of practicing medicine. A year later he wrote an article in defense of vivisection for the journal *Science*. In his last years he read voraciously, especially histories and biographies. "I've got to cultivate my intellect," he told an interviewer on his ninety-fifth birthday. A little less than six months later, on the night of June 7, 1932, he died quietly in his sleep. His obituaries were lavish. None failed to mention his role in the secret operation on Grover Cleveland.

Frances Folsom Cleveland Preston would live to see the Great Depression, the only economic downturn in American history worse than the one derisively named for her first husband. In 1947 she was seated next to Dwight Eisenhower at a formal dinner. Her place card identified her only as Mrs. Thomas Preston. Ike had no idea who she was until they began chatting about Washington. Frances mentioned that she had lived there a long time ago.

"Really?" said Ike. "Where?"

Only then did Frances identify herself as the former First Lady.

Frances died later that year. She was eighty-three. She had been married to Thomas Preston for thirty-four years, twelve more years than she had been married to Grover.

Frances is buried next to Grover in the Princeton cemetery. Their last surviving child, Francis Grover Cleveland, died in 1995 at age ninety-two.

John Erdmann, who had been Joseph Bryant's twenty-nine-year-old assistant at the time of the Cleveland operation, was the last living witness to the events on the *Oneida*. Erdmann enjoyed a long and productive career as a surgeon in New York City. In his later years he traditionally performed an operation on his birthday. (One wonders how his patients felt about this peculiar custom.) On his eighty-sixth birthday in 1950 he removed an appendix. Erdmann would live to see what we would consider the modern antiseptic operating room. In his old age, he enjoyed recounting his role in the Cleveland operation, and he would reflect nostalgically on the folly of it. "We [the surgeons] put our aprons over our street clothes," he told one interviewer, "but we did boil the instruments."

Erdmann died on March 27, 1954—his ninetieth birthday. He did not perform his traditional operation on his final day. His obituaries noted that he had taken part in more than twenty thousand operations in his lifetime—but only one patient was identified by name.

The ultimate fate of the *Oneida* is unknown. Around 1914, Elias Benedict sold the yacht, which was rechristened the *Adelante* and converted into a towboat. During World War I the *Adelante* was commandeered by the U.S. Navy and put into service setting up a network of maritime radio stations along the Maine coast. After the war, it went back into service as a towboat, operating out of New York under the names *John Gulley* and *Salvager*. By 1941, the boat, once one of the grandest yachts in the world and the site of a unique episode in American history, had been abandoned. Presumably it was sold for scrap.

And what became of the tumor that was removed from Grover Cleveland's mouth in 1893? Shortly after the operation it came into the possession of Kasson Gibson, the dentist who fashioned Grover's oral prosthesis. Gibson kept the tumor in a small glass jar filled with a clear preserving fluid. Apparently he stored it in his New York office, a bodily souvenir of his work on the president.

While researching his *Saturday Evening Post* article, W. W. Keen discovered that Gibson still had the tumor, as well as two of the casts Gibson had made of Grover's mouth to prepare the prosthetic devices. At the time, Keen was an active member of the College of Physicians of Philadelphia (not a college in the usual sense, but a private medical society). Keen sent a letter to Gibson urging him to donate the tumor and the casts to the college.

> I spoke to Mrs. Preston about the final disposal of the specimens, etc. and suggested this to her; that as they were of such national interest and as I am going to deposit in the Museum of the College of Physicians of Philadelphia the unusual retractor which we used to draw back the angles of the mouth and expose the seat of the operation . . . it would be desirable that the specimens that you have from the jaw, and, if you are willing, the casts (or duplicates of them) should all be deposited finally with the College of Physicians.

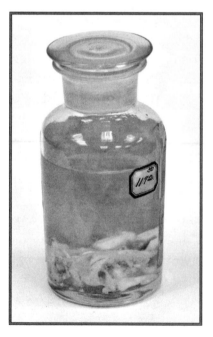

The tumor removed from the mouth of Grover Cleveland in 1893. After the operation, the tumor came into the possession of the dentist Kasson Gibson, who donated it to the College of Physicians of Philadelphia in 1917. MÜTTER MUSEUM OF THE COLLEGE OF PHYSICIANS OF PHILADELPHIA

Gibson agreed to donate the tumor to the college, as well as photographs of the casts. The casts themselves he donated to the New York Academy of Medicine.

On October 3, 1917, Keen presented to the college the tumor, the cheek retractor, and the photographs of the casts, as well as a small laryngeal mirror that was also used in the operation.

The tumor was subsequently put on display in the college's Mütter Museum, where it resides to this day. Named for a nineteenth-century doctor, the Mütter (pronounced MOO-ter) has become a repository for all manner of odd medical specimens, including a piece of John Wilkes Booth's thorax, a section of the brain of Garfield assassin Charles Guiteau, Chief Justice John Marshall's bladder stones, and the Chevalier Jackson Collection, featuring foreign bodies removed from human air and food passages, including bones, pins, hardware, nuts, seeds, teeth, toys, medical instruments, and food.

Grover's tumor is still in the same glass jar it was in when Kasson Gibson donated it to the college in 1917. In the summer of 2010, the tumor sat on a shelf in a large and crowded display case, crammed between a massive ovarian cyst and the skeleton of a twenty-five-year-old Bohemian woman with fused vertebrae. The curatorial text that accompanies the tumor blandly announces:

Tumor—Specimen Removed from the maxillary (upper) left jaw of President Grover Cleveland on July 1st, 1893. 1172.50

The tumor is remarkably well preserved. It looks a bit like a piece of limp cauliflower, though it actually consists of at least ten fragments of tissue and bone, as well as five teeth, including one with a filling—gold, naturally. It's really not much to look at, but for decades this amorphous whitish blob tantalized medical and presidential historians, some of whom had come to question whether Grover Cleveland had suffered from a malignancy at all, or whether his lesion was actually some type of benign tumor. In fact, that blob had the potential to answer a host of lingering questions:

Exactly what kind of tumor was removed from Grover's mouth?

Was it related, as some believe, to an intestinal tumor that eventually killed him?

Was the radical surgery that was performed on Grover the most advisable treatment?

Did Grover have syphilis?

It was this last question that stymied attempts to examine the tumor. As early as 1939, pathologists asked the College of Physicians for permission to conduct tests on the tissue. But the requests were always denied because Grover's children feared the results might reveal that their father suffered from the venereal disease.

In 1967—seventy-four years after the operation—the children finally relented. "My family and I have no objection to having a pathologic examination conducted on the tumor removed from my father's mouth," Grover's elder son Richard wrote in a letter to the college. "I hope that a re-examination of the tumor in the light of present day pathologic knowledge will shed additional light on the true nature of the tumor." If the results were found to be "of a questionable nature," however, the family reserved the right to forbid their publication.

Another eight years passed before the college finally released the tumor for a pathological examination. In 1975, Gonzalo Aponte and Horatio Enterline, eminent Philadelphia pathologists who also sat on the board of the Mütter, were permitted to examine the tumor, "provided that only minimal damage to it would result." Aponte died unexpectedly soon thereafter. He was replaced by John S. J. Brooks, who had only recently completed his residency in pathology. "I guess they needed a gofer," Brooks recalled in a 2010 interview. "I went to the museum and photographed all the fragments of tissue." Brooks also extracted tiny samples from several of the fragments for microscopic examination. This was all done under the careful watch of museum officials, who would not allow the tumor to be removed from the premises. "It was like being back in a high school chemistry class," Brooks remembered.

Brooks and Enterline ultimately determined that the tumor in Grover Cleveland's mouth was a verrucous carcinoma, or VC, a very rare type of cancer that, while technically malignant, grows slowly and does not metastasize. VC accounts for as little as 1 percent of all oral cancers. It's so rare that John Brooks, who is now an esteemed Philadelphia pathologist himself, said he has seen only two other cases in his career besides Grover's.

VC predominantly occurs in the mouths of men between fifty and eighty years of age (Grover was fifty-six), and it often appears in users of snuff and chewing tobacco (Grover's tumor was on the "cigar-chewing side" of his mouth). It is also associated with the use of alcohol. Pathologists grade cancerous tumors on a scale of one to three, with one being the least dangerous. John Brooks estimated that Grover's tumor was "probably about a one-half." "It's almost a benign tumor," Brooks said. If left untreated, however, VC tumors can kill, because they can grow large enough to make eating and breathing impossible.

Grover Cleveland's oral cancer was not, as his doctors believed, exactly the same as Ulysses S. Grant's, which was a more common and more lethal form of squamous cell carcinoma. Brooks and Enterline also concluded that the gelatinous mass removed from Cleveland's antrum, which had so puzzled his doctors, was actually an inflammatory reaction to the tumor—in other words, a kind of infection.

It's not surprising that Grover's doctors were unable to correctly diagnose his tumor. VC wasn't even identified until 1948, when a pathologist named Lauren Ackerman recognized it as a distinct variety of oral cancer. Even today, medical textbooks warn pathologists that VC is very difficult to diagnose, because the tumors closely resemble other, more lethal cancers.

Since VC tumors don't metastasize, Brooks and Enterline also concluded that it was "improbable that the [oral tumor] was the source of Mr. Cleveland's terminal gastrointestinal symptoms," though the "possibility that the former president died of cancer is not eliminated." If

Grover did die of intestinal cancer, it likely had nothing to do with his oral tumor.

Finally, Brooks and Enterline found that Grover did not have syphilis.

The recommended treatment for VC today is "complete surgical excision," so, while Grover's dream team of doctors never knew exactly what kind of tumor was in his mouth, their treatment was certainly appropriate. In fact, they probably overtreated their patient by removing more tissue than was necessary. Today the procedure that Grover Cleveland underwent is known as an intraoral partial maxillectomy, and rather than being fitted with vulcanized rubber prostheses, patients receive reconstructive surgery with bone grafts.

John Brooks and Horatio Enterline published their findings in the March 1980 issue of *Transactions & Studies of the College of Physicians of Philadelphia*. It was not exactly front-page news, though the *Philadelphia Inquirer* ran a small story, noting that the results came "a little late to be of use to Cleveland."

Brooks and Enterline's study concludes, "The character of the original tumor and the skill and aggressiveness of the surgeons combine to explain the successful outcome of the primary illness." Even in 2010, Brooks still marveled at the operation. "I can't believe they did it on a boat," he said, "and they did it in an hour and a half. That's fast! An operation like that today would take a substantial number of hours. It was really one of the most unusual operations in American surgical history."

Brooks wasn't surprised that W. W. Keen decided to publish his account of the operation in the *Saturday Evening Post* instead of a medical journal. "He was a surgeon," Brooks said. "He thought, 'I cured him.' And he wanted to tell the world."

The public's perception of cancer has changed dramatically since 1893. No longer is the word itself avoided in polite company. Nor is cancer considered an automatic death sentence. But the disease has not been conquered, and in some ways it remains the same "dread and mysterious enemy" that E. J. Edwards wrote of in his story about the secret operation on Grover Cleveland. When a large tumor was removed from

President Ronald Reagan's colon in 1985, First Lady Nancy Reagan would not allow the words "cancer" or "malignant" to be used in the statement announcing the operation. Instead, it was announced that the president was undergoing surgery "for removal of a polyp." Two weeks later a small lesion was removed from Reagan's nose and submitted for a biopsy under a false name, "Tracy Malone." Afraid that her husband would be seen as "cancer-prone," Mrs. Reagan ordered the president's press secretary, Larry Speakes, to tell reporters that the scab on the president's nose was caused by the tape used to attach a tube to his nose during his colon surgery.

What followed was reminiscent of the scene inside the barn at Gray Gables ninety-two years earlier, when Dan Lamont insisted President Cleveland was suffering from nothing worse than a bad case of dentistry. At a chaotic press briefing on August 1, 1985, Speakes said the scab on President Reagan's nose was "an irritation from the tape that . . . held the . . . nasogastric tube in place."

"The reporters sensed that something was up," Speakes wrote in his memoir, "and the questions came fast and furious."

> Question: He had a surgical procedure?
>
> Speakes: Yes.
>
> Question: And what was it that was removed?
>
> Speakes: I don't know exactly what it was. It was a skin irritation . . . caused by the tube.
>
> Question: Was it a growth?
>
> Speakes: I don't know. I wouldn't characterize it as a growth. I'd characterize it more as a skin irritation or a gathering of the skin, piling up of the skin or something like that.
>
> Question: You say there will be a biopsy on it?
>
> Speakes: There'll be a routine check of it, yes.
>
> Question: Larry, is the test for cancer? What kind of test is it?
>
> Speakes: I don't know. Just a routine examination, as you would if you had a piece removed from your face.

But unlike the newspapermen in the barn at Gray Gables, these reporters were not willing to give the president the benefit of the doubt.

"I finally acknowledged that what was being done was a biopsy," Speakes later wrote, "although I described the President's health as 'excellent, A-1.'"

After the briefing, Speakes fired off an angry note to the First Lady. "The press questions will not go away and will only become worse if we seek to avoid the obvious question," he wrote. In response, Mrs. Reagan came up with a new cover story: a rogue pimple. In a note to Speakes she wrote, "Why can't we just say—You asked about the Band-Aid on the Pres. nose. He had had a pimple on his nose which he picked at & irritated it."

The White House eventually released a fifty-word statement that omitted the words "cancer" and "biopsy." Speakes, believing his credibility was at stake, pointedly refused to attach his name to the statement. The biopsy revealed that the lesion was a basal cell carcinoma—skin cancer. On August 5, 1985, President Reagan himself finally admitted that he had had a cancerous growth removed—an admission that Grover Cleveland never had to make.

ACKNOWLEDGMENTS

I AM DEEPLY GRATEFUL for all the people who have helped me with this project. My agent, Jane Dystel, believed in it from the beginning. Without her hard work and stellar advice, this book never would have seen the light of day. Thank you, Jane.

Jerry Pohlen, my editor at Chicago Review Press, was, as usual, an absolute joy to work with (even after his basement flooded—twice).

The following institutions assisted me in ways large and small, and each was indispensable: Alexander Mitchell Public Library, Aberdeen, South Dakota; Association of American Medical Colleges; Bowdoin College Library; British Dental Association Dental Museum, London; Centro Studi Americani, Rome; College of Physicians of Philadelphia; Columbia University Libraries, Rare Book and Manuscript Library; Connecticut State Library; District of Columbia Public Library; Free Library of Philadelphia; Frohring Library, John Cabot University, Rome; Georgetown University Library; Greenwich Library, Greenwich, Connecticut; Grover Cleveland Birthplace State Historic Site, Caldwell, New Jersey; Historical Society of the Town of Greenwich, Connecticut; Library of Congress, Law Library of Congress; Library of Congress, Manuscript Reading Room; Library of Congress, Newspaper and Current Periodical Reading Room; Los Angeles Public Library;

Maine Public Broadcasting Network; Marine Museum at Fall River, Massachusetts; Museum of American Finance, New York; New Haven Free Public Library, New Haven, Connecticut; New York Academy of Medicine; New York Public Library; New York University Health Sciences Libraries; Portland Public Library, Portland, Maine; Thomas Jefferson University Archives and Special Collections; United States Navy, Naval Historical Center; United States Senate Historical Office; Van Pelt Library, University of Pennsylvania; and Yale University Library, Manuscripts and Archives.

Special thanks to John S. J. Brooks, M.D., Chair, Department of Pathology, Pennsylvania Hospital, Philadelphia; Anna Dhody and Evi Numen, College of Physicians of Philadelphia; and Gregory N. Prah, M.D., Chief of Anesthesiology, Brattleboro Memorial Hospital, Brattleboro, Vermont.

In the early stages of this project, Gretchen Worden, the director of the Mütter Museum, was especially kind and helpful. She also had a good sense of humor. I was walking through the museum with her one day when I spotted a freeze-dried housecat on display. I asked her if she liked cats. "Of course," she said. "They're wonderful disease vectors!" Almost single-handedly, Gretchen turned the Mütter into a world-class cultural institution. Her death at the age of fifty-six in 2004 was a great loss.

My sister Ann read an early version of the manuscript and offered valuable advice. My brother Jim patiently answered my questions about all things medical. My brother Howard also offered much advice, some of which was actually helpful.

I would be remiss if I neglected to thank William Williams Keen for publishing his story about the operation in 1917, and Frances Folsom Cleveland Preston for allowing him to do so. If not for them, the truth might never have come to light.

Finally, this book would not have been possible without the love and support of my own First Lady, my beautiful and talented wife, the former Miss Allyson McCollum. I've said it before, and I'll say it again: Allyson is the best girl in the world.

CAST OF CHARACTERS

ELIAS C. BENEDICT

Also known as the Commodore, Benedict was a banking magnate and a close friend of Grover Cleveland. It was on his yacht, the *Oneida*, that the secret operation on Cleveland took place on July 1, 1893.

JOSEPH BRYANT

A prominent New York surgeon and the Cleveland family's physician, Bryant assembled the dream team of surgeons that operated on the president. Bryant was also the lead surgeon during the operation.

FRANCES CLEVELAND

The youngest First Lady in history, Frances Folsom married Grover Cleveland when she was just twenty-one years old. At the time of the operation on her husband, Frances was pregnant with the couple's second child.

GROVER CLEVELAND

Twice elected president of the United States, Cleveland was diagnosed with cancer early in his second term. At the time the country was in the midst of an economic crisis that came to be known as the Panic of 1893.

CHARLES A. DANA
The publisher of the *New York Sun*, Dana hired E. J. Edwards in 1879. His great rival was *New York World* publisher Joseph Pulitzer.

ELISHA JAY (E. J.) EDWARDS
At the *New York Sun* and, later, the *Philadelphia Press*, Edwards established himself as one of the great reporters of his generation. Writing under the pen name Holland, he broke the story of the president's secret operation.

JOHN ERDMANN
A protégé of Joseph Bryant, Erdmann was the youngest member of the surgical team that operated on the president. At the time of the operation, he was just twenty-nine.

KASSON GIBSON
A New York dentist and prosthodontist, Gibson fashioned a vulcanized-rubber prosthetic device to plug the hole in Cleveland's mouth after the operation. This restored the president's normal appearance and speaking voice.

FERDINAND HASBROUCK
A dentist who was also an experienced anesthetist, Hasbrouck extracted teeth and administered nitrous oxide during the operation on the president. His missed appointment the day after the operation would have profound consequences.

EDWARD JANEWAY
An accomplished surgeon, Janeway monitored the president's vital signs during the operation.

WILLIAM WILLIAMS (W. W.) KEEN
Perhaps the most famous surgeon in the country at the time, Keen assisted Joseph Bryant during the operation.

DANIEL LAMONT

A former newspaper reporter, Lamont was Cleveland's private secretary in his first administration and his secretary of war in his second. He also acted as the president's unofficial press secretary.

ALEXANDER K. MCCLURE

As publisher of the *Philadelphia Times*, McClure spearheaded a campaign to discredit E. J. Edwards and his story about the secret operation in the rival *Philadelphia Press*.

ROBERT LINCOLN O'BRIEN

As Cleveland's private secretary in his second administration, O'Brien helped Daniel Lamont orchestrate a cover-up of the secret operation.

ROBERT M. O'REILLY

As the White House physician, O'Reilly helped organize the secret operation, during which he administered ether.

JOSEPH PULITZER

As publisher of the *New York World*, Pulitzer was an early practitioner of yellow journalism.

CHARLES EMORY SMITH

As publisher of the *Philadelphia Press*, Smith lured E. J. Edwards away from the *New York Sun* in 1889. It was in the *Press* that Edwards's explosive account of the operation was published.

ADLAI STEVENSON

The grandfather of the 1952 and 1956 Democratic presidential nominee of the same name, Stevenson was Cleveland's vice president in his second administration. Unlike the president, Stevenson was a silverite and opposed repeal of the Silver Purchase Act.

SOURCES

THERE WERE CERTAIN CHALLENGES in researching and writing a century-old story that was never meant to be told. For one thing, the main characters are long dead. Fortunately, however, many of them bequeathed their papers to institutions that have made them available to the public. These papers were invaluable to my research:

Grover Cleveland (papers held by the Library of Congress)

Stephen Crane (Columbia University Library)

Kasson C. Gibson (New York Academy of Medicine)

Charles S. Hamlin (Library of Congress)

William Williams Keen (College of Physicians of Philadelphia)

Daniel S. Lamont (Library of Congress)

Robert Lincoln O'Brien (Library of Congress)

Richard Olney (Library of Congress)

Most valuable were the papers of William Williams Keen. In addition to being a prolific writer, Dr. Keen was also an inveterate saver. He meticulously collected correspondence and clippings related to the operation in a large scrapbook, an irreplaceable resource that was crucial to my research.

Unfortunately, Elisha Jay Edwards's papers have not survived. One summer morning in 1908, children playing with matches ignited a fire that engulfed much of Greenwich, Connecticut. Miraculously, no one was killed, but the blaze consumed a dozen homes, including E. J.'s. A lifetime of notes, letters, and clippings went up in flames, including the priceless records of his reporting on the Cleveland operation and the Sugar Trust scandal.

With the help of the archivists at Yale University, however, I was able to piece together Edwards's biography. Especially helpful were the records contained in his alumni files, as well as his yearbooks and class reunion books.

My account is also based on contemporaneous newspaper reports. I scoured dozens of papers on microfilm, in bound volumes, and, through the miracle of the Internet, online in the comfort of my home. These papers are cited in the text. I am deeply indebted to the newspaper reporters, mostly anonymous, whose work in the late nineteenth century made mine in the early twenty-first much easier. Their names may be lost to history, but their work continues to inform us.

BIBLIOGRAPHY

Armitage, Charles H. *Grover Cleveland as Buffalo Knew Him*. Buffalo, NY: Buffalo Evening News, 1926.

Barber, Douglas. "The Pawn in the Gambit." *British Dental Journal*, November 1987.

Barton, Clara. *The Red Cross in Peace and War*. Meriden, CT: Journal Publishing Company, 1912.

Bennett, A. E. "The Secret Surgical Operation on President Cleveland." *The Pharos of Alpha Omega Alpha*, October 1975.

Berryman, John. *Stephen Crane: A Critical Biography*. New York: Cooper Square Press, 2001.

Blair, Edward. *Leadville: Colorado's Magic City*. Boulder, CO: Pruett Publishing, 1980.

Boller, Paul F., Jr. *Presidential Inaugurations*. New York: Harcourt, 2001.

Bollet, Alfred Jay. "Grover Cleveland's Secret Cancer." *Resident & Staff Physician*, August 1979.

Brands, H. W. *The Reckless Decade: America in the 1890s*. New York: St. Martin's Press, 1995.

Brodsky, Alyn. *Grover Cleveland: A Study in Character*. New York: St. Martin's Press, 2000.

Brooks, John S. J., Horatio T. Enterline, and Gonzalo E. Aponte. "The Final Diagnosis of President Cleveland's Lesion." *Transactions & Studies of the College of Physicians of Philadelphia*, March 1980.

Brooks, John S. J. "President Cleveland's Curative Surgery for Oral Carcinoma." *Contemporary Surgery*, January 1982.

Brown, Henry Collins. *In the Golden Nineties*. Hastings-on-Hudson, NY: Valentine's Manual, 1928.

Bumgarner, John R. *The Health of the Presidents: The 41 United States Presidents through 1993 from a Physician's Point of View*. Jefferson, NC: McFarland & Company, 1994.

Butler, Fracelia. "President Cleveland Scoops the Press." *American Mercury*, January 1954.

Carlson, Eric. "Oral Cancer and United States Presidents." *Journal of Oral and Maxillofacial Surgery*, February 2002.

Cashman, Sean Dennis. *America in the Gilded Age: From the Death of Lincoln to the Rise of Theodore Roosevelt*. New York: New York University Press, 1984.

Chace, James. *1912: Wilson, Roosevelt, Taft & Debs—The Election That Changed the Country*. New York: Simon & Schuster, 2004.

Churchill, Allen. *Park Row: A Vivid Re-creation of Turn of the Century Newspaper Days*. New York: Rinehart & Company, 1958.

DeGregorio, William A. *The Complete Book of U.S. Presidents*. New York: Barricade Books, 1993.

Deppisch, Ludwig M. "President Cleveland's Secret Operation: The Effect of the Office upon the Care of the President." *The Pharos of Alpha Omega Alpha*, Summer 1995.

———. *The White House Physician: A History from Washington to George W. Bush*. Jefferson, NC: McFarland & Company, 2007.

Drabelle, Dennis. *Mile-High Fever: Silver Mines, Boom Towns, and High Living on the Comstock Lode*. New York: St. Martin's Press, 2009.

Edwards, Elisha Jay. *American Achievements*. New York: London Press Association, 1926.

———. *The Free Silver Conspiracy (16 to 1): A True Story*. Philadelphia: Hubbard Publishing, 1896.

———. "The Great Railroad Builders." *Munsey's Magazine*, February 1903.

_____. "'Holland' Tells How He Got News of 'Press' Beat." *Philadelphia Press*, September 26, 1917.

_____. "The Personal Force of Cleveland." *McClure's Magazine*, November 1893.

_____. "The Two Broken Appointments that Gave the Country a Sensation." *The Evening Mail Magazine* (New York), October 6, 1917.

Ferrell, Robert H. *Ill-Advised: Presidential Health and Public Trust.* Columbia, MO: University of Missouri Press, 1992.

Flexner, Abraham. *Medical Education in the United States and Canada.* New York: Carnegie Foundation, 1910.

Ford, Henry Jones. *The Cleveland Era: A Chronicle of the New Order in Politics.* New Haven: Yale University Press, 1919.

Geary, James W. *We Need Men: The Union Draft in the Civil War.* DeKalb, IL: Northern Illinois University Press, 1991.

Graff, Henry F. *Grover Cleveland.* New York: Times Books, 2002.

Herskowitz, Linda. "1893 Presidential Tumor Analyzed at Last." *Philadelphia Inquirer*, January 10, 1981.

Hoang, Hoat M., and J. Patrick O'Leary. "President Grover Cleveland's Secret Operation." *American Surgeon*, August 1997.

Hotchner, A. E. "Jaws of Death." *George*, August 1997.

Hudson, William C. *Random Recollections of an Old Political Reporter.* New York: Cupples & Leon Company, 1911.

James, W. W. Keen, ed. *Keen of Philadelphia: The Collected Memoirs of William Williams Keen Jr.* Dublin, NH: William L. Bauhan, 2002.

Jeffers, H. Paul. *An Honest President: The Life and Presidencies of Grover Cleveland.* New York: HarperCollins, 2000.

Keen, William W. *The Surgical Operations on President Cleveland in 1893 Together with Six Additional Papers of Reminiscences.* Philadelphia: J. B. Lippincott Company, 1928.

LaFrance, Marston. "A Few Facts about Stephen Crane and 'Holland.'" *American Literature*, May 1965.

Larson, Merlin. "Grover Cleveland's Request." *California Society of Anesthesiologists Bulletin*, Winter 2008.

Lindsey, Almont. *The Pullman Strike: The Story of a Unique Experiment and of a Great Labor Upheaval.* Chicago: University of Chicago Press, 1942.

Lynch, Denis Tilden. *Grover Cleveland: A Man Four-Square*. New York: Horace Liveright, 1932.

MacMahon, Edward B., and Leonard Curry. *Medical Cover-Ups in the White House*. Washington, DC: Farragut Publishing, 1987.

Maranto, Robert, and David Schultz. *A Short History of the United States Civil Service*. Lanham, MD: University Press of America, 1991.

Marscher, Bill, and Fran Marscher. *The Great Sea Island Storm of 1893*. Macon, GA: Mercer University Press, 2004.

Martin, John Stuart. "When the President Disappeared." *American Heritage*, October 1957.

McClure, Alexander K. *Colonel Alexander K. McClure's Recollections of Half a Century*. Salem, MA: Salem Press Company, 1902.

McCutcheon, Marc. *Everyday Life in the 1800s: A Guide for Writers, Students and Historians*. Cincinnati: Writer's Digest Books, 1993.

McElroy, Robert. *Grover Cleveland: The Man and the Statesman*. New York: Harper & Brothers, 1923.

Merrill, Horace Samuel. *Bourbon Leader: Grover Cleveland and the Democratic Party*. Boston: Little, Brown and Company, 1957.

Miller, Joseph M. "Stephen Grover Cleveland." *Surgery, Gynecology and Obstetrics*, October 1961.

Mills, Stacey E., Michael J. Gaffey, and Henry F. Frierson Jr. *Tumors of the Upper Aerodigestive Tract and Ear*. Washington, DC: Armed Forces Institute of Pathology, 2000.

Morreels, Charles L. "New Historical Information on the Cleveland Operations." *Surgery*, September 1967.

Morris, James McGrath. *Pulitzer: A Life in Politics, Print, and Power*. New York: Harper, 2010.

Moses, John B., and Wilbur Cross. "When the President Vanished." *Journal of the California Dental Association*, April 1999.

Mott, Frank Luther. *American Journalism: A History of Newspapers in the United States through 260 Years: 1690 to 1950*. New York: Macmillan, 1950.

Nelson, Henry Loomis. "A Day at Gray Gables." *Harper's Weekly*, July 23, 1892.

Nevins, Allan. *Grover Cleveland: A Study in Courage*. New York: Dodd, Mead & Company, 1934.

————, ed. *Letters of Grover Cleveland 1850–1908*. Boston: Houghton Mifflin Company, 1933.

Nichols, Jeannette Paddock. "The Politics and Personalities of Silver Repeal in the United States Senate." *American Historical Review*, October 1935.

O'Brien, Robert Lincoln. "Keeping a Nation's Secret 24 Years." *Boston Herald*, September 30, 1917.

Patterson, James T. *The Dread Disease: Cancer and Modern American Culture*. Cambridge, MA: Harvard University Press, 1987.

Perry, Mark. *Grant and Twain: The Story of an American Friendship*. New York: Random House, 2004.

Peterkin, Allan. *One Thousand Beards: A Cultural History of Facial Hair*. Vancouver: Arsenal Pulp Press, 2001.

Pollard, James E. *The Presidents and the Press, Truman to Johnson*. Washington, DC: Public Affairs Press, 1964.

Renehan, Andrew, and John C. Lowry. "The Oral Tumours of Two American Presidents: What if They Were Alive Today?" *Journal of the Royal Society of Medicine*, July 1995.

"The Right of a Newsman to Refrain from Divulging the Sources of His Information." *Virginia Law Review*, Volume 36, 1950.

Ritter, Gretchen. *Goldbugs and Greenbacks: The Antimonopoly Tradition and the Politics of Finance in America, 1865–1896*. New York: Cambridge University Press, 1997.

Robson, J. Stuart. "The Day a President Disappeared." *Dental Historian*, January 2007.

Rosenhouse, Leo. "President Cleveland's Secret Surgery." *Private Practice*, October 1974.

Rothstein, William G. *American Medical Schools and the Practice of Medicine: A History*. New York: Oxford University Press, 1987.

Rutkow, Ira M. *American Surgery: An Illustrated History*. Philadelphia: Lippincott-Raven, 1998.

Seale, William. *The President's House: A History*. Baltimore: Johns Hopkins University Press, 2008.

Seelig, M. G. "Cancer and Politics: The Operation on Grover Cleveland." *Surgery, Gynecology and Obstetrics*, September 1947.

Smith, Richard Norton. "'The President Is Fine' and Other Historical Lies." *Columbia Journalism Review*, September/October 2001.

Speakes, Larry. *Speaking Out: The Reagan Presidency from Inside the White House*. New York: Charles Scribner's Sons, 1988.

Steeples, Douglas, and David O. Whitten. *Democracy in Desperation: The Depression of 1893*. Westport, CT: Greenwood Press, 1998.

"The Surgical Operations on President Cleveland." *Physicians' Times Magazine*, circa 1928 (undated clipping on file at the College of Physicians of Philadelphia).

Truax, Rhoda. *Joseph Lister: Father of Modern Surgery*. Indianapolis: Bobbs-Merrill, 1944.

Tullai, Martin D. "How Grover Cleveland Concealed from Nation His Cancer Operation." *Buffalo News*, March 13, 1994.

United States Congress. *Congressional Record*. 52nd Congress, 2nd Session, 1894.

Voynick, Stephen M. *Leadville: A Miner's Epic*. Missoula, MT: Mountain Press, 1984.

Walter, Dave. *Today Then: America's Best Minds Look 100 Years into the Future on the Occasion of the 1893 World's Columbian Exposition*. Helena, MT: American & World Geographic Publishing, 1992.

Weatherford, Richard M., ed. *Stephen Crane: The Critical Heritage*. Boston: Routledge and Kegan Paul, 1973.

Welch, Richard E. *The Presidencies of Grover Cleveland*. Lawrence, KS: University Press of Kansas, 1988.

Wertheim, Stanley, and Paul Sorrentino, eds. *The Correspondence of Stephen Crane*. New York: Columbia University Press, 1988.

Whitcomb, John, and Claire Whitcomb. *Real Life in the White House: 200 Years of Daily Life at America's Most Famous Residence*. New York: Routledge, 2000.

INDEX

Also by Matthew Algeo

HARRY TRUMAN'S
Excellent Adventure
The True Story of a Great American Road Trip

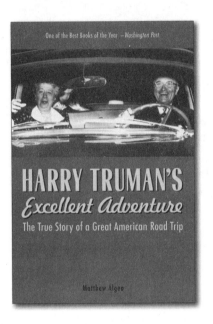

One of the Best Books of 2009 —*Washington Post*

"Utterly likeable." —Christopher Buckley

"An engaging account." —*Wall Street Journal*

"[An] enchanting glimpse into a much simpler age."
—*Library Journal*

Paperback • 978-1-56976-707-8
Includes a new afterword from the author

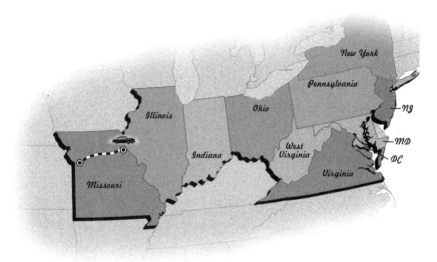

Hannibal, Missouri,
June 19, 1953

On Friday, June 19, 1953, Harry skipped his morning constitutional and devoted himself to packing. He and Bess planned to hit the road that morning—and they would not travel light. Harry would fill the New Yorker with eleven suitcases before he was finished, the luggage spilling out of the trunk and onto the backseat. Most people hate packing, but Harry Truman, true to his obsessive nature, relished the task. "He prided himself on being an expert packer," his daughter, Margaret, remembered, "and he was."

Around 7:15, Harry and Bess climbed into the big black car. Harry slowly backed it through the narrow gate at the end of the driveway and onto Van Horn Road (soon to be renamed Truman Road). He had already scraped some chrome off the car backing through the gate, a process he likened to "the camel and the needle's eye." They drove the half-block up Van Horn, turned right onto Delaware Street, went about a mile, then turned right onto U.S. Highway 24. This they would follow 166 miles east to Monroe City, where they would pick up Highway 36.

A crude early version of air-conditioning was an option on the New Yorker in 1953, but Harry's didn't have it. (He never much saw the need for AC.) Missouri was in the grips of a heat wave, and the mercury would top 100 in much of the state that day. In Kansas City it hit 102. So the Trumans rode with the windows rolled all the way down, Harry with both hands on the wheel, Bess resting her elbow on the open window frame. They were, as usual, impeccably dressed: Harry wore a white suit, Bess a rayon print dress. Harry did make one small concession to the heat, however: he drove in his shirtsleeves, his jacket hanging from a hook above the left rear window.

As Independence faded in his rearview mirror, Harry Truman might have been the happiest man in Missouri, if not all forty-eight states. He loved to drive. Back when he was a county judge, he'd driven thousands of miles touring county courthouses from Colorado to New York before the construction of the new courthouse in Independence. When he ran for the Senate in 1934, he campaigned by car, crisscrossing the Show-Me State in

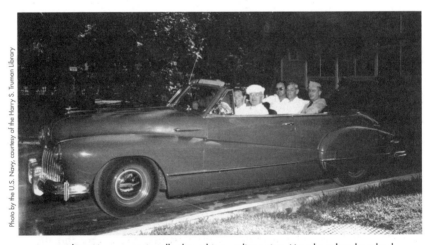

As president, Harry occasionally drove his own limousine. Here he takes the wheel during a vacation in Key West in 1946.

his shiny new Plymouth. He enjoyed it so much, he said he felt like he was on vacation. As a senator, he drove thousands of miles investigating fraud and waste on military bases throughout the South and Midwest and, of course, he regularly drove between Independence and Washington. He always preferred the freedom of the road to the plush confines of a Pullman car. Even when he was president, he would occasionally take the wheel of his limo, much to the consternation of his Secret Service agents.

Driving not only satisfied his need to keep moving; it also helped him gauge the country's mood. "You have to get around and listen to what people are saying," he said.

He fancied himself an excellent driver, naturally, but in reality, riding shotgun with Harry Truman could be a hair-raising adventure. As his longtime friend Mize Peters once told an interviewer, rather diplomatically, "I have driven with him when I was a little uneasy."

By far his biggest vice was speed. Bess was right: Harry drove too fast.

On July 6, 1947, Truman drove a White House limousine back to Washington from an engagement in Charlottesville, Virginia. His passengers included Treasury Secretary John W. Snyder and Admiral William Leahy. Reporters clocked Truman at speeds approaching sixty-five miles per hour on country roads where the posted speed limit was fifty. When the *Richmond Times-Dispatch* reported the transgression, Truman responded with one of his legendary "longhand spasms." "The pace was set by a capable, efficient State Policeman, in a State Police car," he wrote in an angry letter to the paper. "I could not have exceeded the Virginia speed law if I had desired to do so—which I did not." He never sent the letter.

There is no evidence that he was ever charged with a traffic violation, but Harry Truman's driving record was not perfect. On Sunday, March 27, 1938, he was driving home from Washington with Bess and Margaret when he blew through a stop sign at a busy intersection in Hagerstown, Maryland. Another car plowed into them. Truman's car—a brand-new Plymouth—rolled several times and was totaled. Nobody in either car was seriously injured. "It was almost a miracle that we escaped alive," Margaret remembered. Truman claimed the stop sign was obscured by a parked car. No citations were issued, but a judge ordered Truman to pay the other driver ninety dollars for damages. In his later years, Harry's escapades behind the

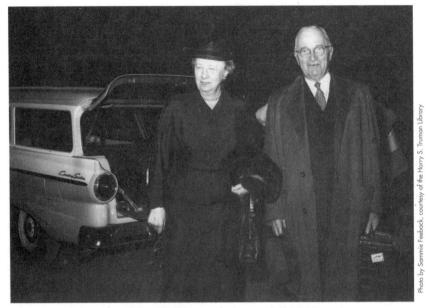

Harry and Bess on a trip in 1957. The Trumans were one of those lucky couples who travel well together, though Bess always thought Harry drove too fast.

wheel would become the stuff of legend in Independence. As the *Kansas City Star* once put it, Truman navigated the corridors of power more gracefully than the streets of his hometown. Mostly he was involved in fender benders. Usually he offered the other driver cash to pay for repairs—reportedly so Bess wouldn't find out. (At least one driver refused the money, preferring to preserve his dent as a unique kind of presidential souvenir.) "I'd hear the fellows down at the filling station talk about Mr. Truman out driving around," remembered Sue Gentry, associate editor of the *Independence Examiner.* "They'd say, 'You'd better watch him—he's getting a little wild out there.'"

Bess, of course, had made Harry promise that he would drive no faster than fifty-five miles per hour, even though the speed limit on many highways at the time was sixty or sixty-five—and in some places there were no limits at all. (In Missouri, for example, drivers were merely required to maintain a "reasonable and prudent" speed.) But, owing to his lead foot, Harry found it almost impossible to keep that promise. Just a few miles outside Independence, Bess turned to him and said, "What does the speedometer say?"

"Fifty-five," Harry answered.

"Do you think I'm losing my eyesight? Slow down!"

Harry obeyed, and soon everything else on the road was passing the decelerated Trumans. "Not only that," Harry remembered, "but since we were going so slowly, they had a chance to look us over. Pretty soon the shouted greetings started: 'Hi, Harry!' 'Where you going, Harry?' 'Hey! Wasn't that Harry Truman?'"

"Well," Harry said to Bess, a bit of I-told-you-so in his voice, "there goes our incognito—and I don't mean a part of the car."

About an hour after leaving Independence, they crossed the Missouri River near the town of Waverly. When Harry had first proposed the trip, Bess had had her doubts. But now that they were on the road, those doubts melted away in the withering heat. On the bridge over the Missouri, Bess turned to Harry. "Isn't it good to be on our own again," she said, "doing as we please as we did in the old Senate days?"

"I said that I thought it was grand," Harry remembered, "and that I hoped we'd do as we pleased from that time on."